Schedules

for

Clinical

Assessment

in

Neuropsychiatry

Version 2

GLOSSARY

Differential definitions of SCAN items
and commentary on the SCAN manual

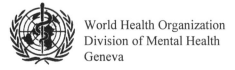

World Health Organization
Division of Mental Health
Geneva

D0904022

ACKNOWLEDGEMENTS

The development of SCAN was funded by NIH,WHO, the Field Trial Centers, and the Institutes employing individual contributors.

World Health Organization: *N Sartorius, TB Üstün*

NIH: *D Regier (NIMH), J Blaine(NIDA), B Grant and L Towle(NIAAA).*

Glossary editors: *T Babor, P Bebbington, A Bertelsen, T Brugha, S Chatterji, M Isaac, AJ Romanoski, AY Tien, TB Üstün, LG Wing, JK Wing.*

Chief Editor: *JK Wing*

Acknowledgements to the work of centers and individuals who helped in the development of particular components of SCAN will be found in the SCAN text.

Contents of SCAN Glossary

General introduction to the SCAN system

DEVELOPMENT AND BASIC PRINCIPLES

The SCAN system (Schedules for Clinical Assessment in Neuropsychiatry) is a set of instruments and manuals aimed at assessing, measuring and classifying the psychopathology and behavior associated with the major psychiatric disorders of adult life. The SCAN text has 3 components: the tenth edition of the Present State Examination (PSE10), the Item Group Checklist (IGC) and the Clinical History Schedule (CHS). PSE10 itself has two parts. Part I covers somatoform, dissociative, anxiety, depressive and bipolar disorders, and problems associated with appetite, alcohol and other substance use. There is also a screen for Part II conditions. Part II covers psychotic and cognitive disorders and observed abnormalities of speech, affect and behavior.

The SCAN system contains two other essential elements: the Glossary of differential definitions and CATEGO, a set of computer programs for processing SCAN data and providing output.

Data from the schedules can be entered into CATEGO in a variety of ways: on the SCAN Schedules themselves, on SCAN Coding Sheets, and into a computer program.

Output from CATEGO is presented as a series of options, including a range of profiles of symptom and IGC scores, an Index of Definition, ICD-10 and DSM categories, a prediagnostic profile of categories, and a list of items rated present.

There are two manuals; one is a Training Pack for SCAN training centers, the other a Reference Manual for a more general readership and SCAN users.

These contain details concerning the development of SCAN, instructions as to its use, and the results of international trials of feasibility and reliability. The SCAN Glossary is presented in a ring-bound format for ease of use with the SCAN Manual.

In its complete form, the SCAN text is intended for use only by clinicians with an adequate knowledge of psychopathology who have taken a course at a WHO-designated SCAN training center. A shortened version of Part One of PSE10 can be used (e.g. in two-stage population surveys, as with the equivalent version of PSE9) by lay interviewers trained in these centers.

SCAN represents the latest stage in a 30-year line of development that began in the late 1950s. PSE9 was the first of the series to be published, following 15 years of work on earlier versions, including two large multicenter international projects - the US-UK Diagnostic Project (1972) and the International Pilot Study of Schizophrenia (IPSS; WHO, 1973). PSE9 consists of only 140 items, compared to the 500-600 of PSE7 and PSE8. It has been widely used, as evidenced by its translation into 35 or more languages, but many users have regretted that the longer preceding editions were withdrawn; they would have preferred a choice, which is now provided by PSE10.

The principles underlying the PSE have changed very little during these developments but they have gradually been applied to a broader range of disorders, have come to incorporate more and more aspects of the clinical history and, through the use of an increasingly complex technology, have been preserved without loss of the basic clinical bottom-up approach and user friendliness. An understanding of the history is therefore a useful basis for an appreciation of SCAN. The SCAN Reference Manual provides an overview. A brief bibliography is appended at the end of this Glossary.

The central principle of the PSE is that the interview, although substantially structured, retains the features of a clinical examination. The aim of the interviewer is to discover which of a comprehensive list of phenomena have been present during a designated period of time and with what degree of severity. The items listed are differentially defined in this Glossary, with which the interviewer is expected to be closely familiar. The examination is therefore based on a process of matching the respondent's behavior and description of subjective experiences against the clinical definitions provided.

Applying the central principle means that a rich data base of differentially-defined clinical phenomena forms the core of SCAN. Numerous classifying algorithms can be applied to generate 'diagnoses' according to the criteria of schools that provide sufficiently operational rules. Two of these (ICD, and DSM since its third revision) have won wide international acceptance. But any other set of rules can be applied. A virtue of SCAN is that its clinical database has not been constructed solely in accordance with any one nosology.

"The flexibility of this approach, the incorporation of detailed cross-examination, which allows changes in the order and wording of questions according to the way the interview is going, the freedom of the clinician to pursue some lines of enquiry while cutting off others, the fact that the examiner and not the patient makes the judgement as to whether a symptom is present, do not seriously impair the reliability of the procedure" (Wing et al, 1967). This statement was based on experience with the third to the fifth editions of the PSE and it still holds good.

PSE10

Preparations for a tenth edition of the PSE were started in 1980, in anticipation of the tenth edition of the ICD. The major emphasis of correspondents was on broadening the content, both by returning to the larger item-pool of PSE7 and PSE8, and by adding new sections to cover somatoform, dissociative and eating disorders, alcohol and drug misuse, and cognitive impairments. A second suggestion was that an extra rating point was needed to extend the 0-1-2 scales of severity used for most PSE9 items, allowing a mild or 'sub-clinical' level to be used, particularly in population surveys. A third, very obvious, requirement was for a better system for rating episodes of disorder, adding other information relevant to the history and to the causes of disorder, and processing all the information by means of one set of computer programs. The publication and widespread use of DSM-III and later its revised version, DSM-III-R (APA, 1987), meant that the latter and, perhaps more usefully, DSM-IV (APA, 1994), required clinical supplements. Version Two of SCAN incorporates changes brought about by DSM-IV.

This work has been taken forward by a Task Force on Psychiatric Assessment Instruments, established within the framework of a joint WHO/NIH project aimed at improving the accuracy and reliability of measurement and classification of psychiatric disorders (Jablensky et al, 1983). Apart from SCAN, two other instruments have been sponsored by the Task Force. One is the Composite International Diagnostic Interview (CIDI: Robins et al, 1988) which is designed for use by lay interviewers in population surveys. The other is the International Personality Disorder Examination (IPDE).

An early version of SCAN was used in a study of the service needs of long term attenders at day hospitals and day centers in Camberwell, south-east London (Brugha et al, 1988). This provided a severe test of the historical capacities of SCAN, since the attenders had been in contact with services for an average of 17 years and nearly half did not have conditions that could be diagnosed from a present state interview alone. The results were satisfactory in this respect.

Field trials of the third (February 1988) draft of SCAN were undertaken under the auspices of WHO, after key participants from 20 centers, in 14 countries, had been trained in London. The text was translated into all the local languages, based on the principle that it was more important to translate the concepts than the words. Independent back-translation of the key items was used as a check. Extra trials were undertaken of sections that were not sufficiently tested in the main series because of lack of numbers. These included the eating, cognitive, and alcohol and substance use sections. The results, and detailed reports from the Centers, indicate that feasibility and reliability were fully up to the standards reported for the earlier editions. The practical comments of participating interviewers were invaluable during the innumerable textual revisions of the past five years.

As part of the preparation of SCAN Version 2, incorporating changes necessitated by DSM-IV, further field trials have been carried out providing data on the cross cultural comparability of items on use of alcohol and drugs beyond prescription.

THE PURPOSE OF THE SCAN SYSTEM

The purpose of the SCAN system is to provide comprehensive, accurate and technically specifiable means of describing and classifying psychiatric phenomena, in order to make comparisons.

Training in SCAN techniques provides a common clinical language in which to compare and contrast the experiences and behavior of patients, to consider the usage of different clinical schools in relation to a common reference system, to compare epidemiological and public health data more precisely, and to make the results of scientific research readily available for replication between centers.

CLINICAL CROSS-EXAMINATION

The function of the Glossary is to support the process of clinical cross-examination, which is the central method of obtaining information about the respondent's subjective experiences. Training in the differential definitions provides the examiner with a set of 'item concepts', which are matched against the respondent's descriptions. Only when the description matches the concept does the examiner make the rating. This process helps to eliminate syndromal, diagnostic and other biases, misunderstandings, and 'yea-saying'.

Considerable training and experience is needed before the probe system in the SCAN text can be used flexibly enough in close conjunction with the Glossary to ensure that the ratings most accurately fit the phenomena.

A full description of the technique is given in the Reference Manual and the Training Pack.

COVERAGE OF SCAN

Sections 1-25 of SCAN (PSE10) covers the symptoms and signs of disorders in subchapters F0-F5 of ICD-10 and their equivalents in DSM. Some Sections have optional Checklists attached, which cover items related to disorders that require specific time relationships, for example to psychosocial trauma, as in the stress and adjustment disorders. Other Checklists allow a more extended list of items to be rated than is provided in the main text; for example the extra list of somatoform symptoms, **2.080-2.135**. Optional Checklist items, which include items not already existing elsewhere, are not defined in the Glossary.

SCAN REFERENCE MANUAL

The reference manual is published in book form (Wing *et al.*, 1995. It contains an account of the history and development of SCAN from beginnings in the second half of the 1950s. Chapters are devoted to the aims, the principles and the techniques of SCAN, the results of international field trials, and the varieties of computer output.

SCAN TRAINING PACK

The Glossary is one element in the SCAN Training Pack, which also contains materials for SCAN Training Centers, trainers and trainees. The pack provides a comprehensive introduction to the SCAN text, the Glossary, and the computer programs (including a new SCAN computer program running in Microsoft Windows (tm)), with instructions for their use, materials for SCAN Training Courses, and recommendations concerning the duties of Training Centers. The use of these materials is described in a document obtainable from the Division of Mental Health, World Health Organization, Geneva.

The Glossary is the most important component of SCAN. Extensive experience has demonstrated that it is possible for virtually all clinicians to apply the definitions, even if they would not themselves agree with some of them. The point of using SCAN is not to ensure uniformity of thought but to provide a reference system against which to make comparisons for clinical, educational and research purposes. The Instruction Manual and the Training Pack develop this central principle.

Nearly all clinical items in PSE10 contain a brief definition in the text. Those that involve clinical cross-examination (see below for a description of this method of interviewing) are provided with a list of probes to elicit relevant information from the respondent, and instructions for numerical rating. The Glossary definition is usually more detailed and provides reasons for excluding other possible symptoms. All those who use SCAN should know and be able to apply these differential definitions.

The SCAN Glossary has been developed from that of PSE9, in the light of the accumulated experience of users. The main content of the definitions of equivalent items remains the same, though there is often some elaboration or clarification. Information from the text of ICD-10, its Diagnostic Criteria for Research (DCR), and DSM-III-R and DSM-IV, has also been incorporated where appropriate.

Most 'technical' items in SCAN, such as those dealing with dates, causal attributions, predominance of certain symptom types over others, specific time relationships during the course, etc., also have an explanatory text. The Glossary is therefore not only a dictionary but a brief instruction manual for SCAN. It should be consulted whenever a problem arises that cannot be answered from the SCAN text.

SCAN software is available for use on IBM-compatible desktop or laptop computers. The computer program runs in Microsoft Windows (tm) with a graphical interface. The program displays the SCAN Manual in a window and allows rapid navigation through the manual by Part, Section, and Item numbers. The Glossary is displayed in a window and is automatically linked to the active Manual item, so that information about a particular item is always present. The Glossary can be appended to by the user (in a different font) to assist in further standardization for research purposes. The program also allows an infinite number of episodes to be rated, useful for repeated assessment of an individual, and each item episode can be dated for onset and offset separately from other items. The program displays the ICD-10 and DSM-IV diagnostic algorithms with graphical indicators of relevant SCAN items and their rated values. The computer program can be obtained from WHO/Division of Mental Health or from the SCAN Training and Reference Centers.

TERMINOLOGY

The Glossary contains differential definitions of aspects of experience or behavior that are common among people referred for a specialist psychiatric opinion. Each aspect is allocated an item in the SCAN text, with a unique item-number and item-name. The corresponding definitions are listed in the Glossary in numerical order. 'Items' represent subjectively described 'symptoms' or 'signs' observed in behavior. Symptoms and signs are sometimes referred to as 'phenomena'. (Users of SCAN Version One should note the extensive renumbering of items in Version Two).

These terms might suggest that the items are linked to theories of cause or pathology, and therefore that SCAN items might represent symptoms and signs of diseases. Such hypotheses are not part of the structure of SCAN. A central principle is that phenomena are rated on their own merit, irrespective of any theory about the way they cluster, their causes or their psychosocial or biological nature. It is only in this way that a comprehensive clinical picture can be obtained, on which classifying and/or dimensional rules of various kinds can operate. No particular set of rules should be allowed to influence decisions as to whether any symptom or sign is present. Terms like 'neurotic', 'affective', 'psychotic' and 'organic' are used descriptively, in the same spirit.

There are items where the examiner can make an attribution about pathology or aetiology or relationship to other phenomena, but these are clinical judgements required by rule-based diagnostic systems such as ICD-10 and DSM-IV, not specifications by the SCAN system. As an option, a scale to code attributions of etiology is included in Version 2 of the SCAN. Codes can be entered in boxes with dashed lines below the standard episode rating boxes. The rating of '6' in Scale I in Version 1 of the SCAN has been removed, in order to emphasize rating of phenomenology irrespective of etiology. The terminology of symptoms and signs is used for convenience only. For research purposes, new rating boxes have been added to code etiology attributions if desired. This approach is not fully tested for reliability and validity and is optional.

In Version 1 'Traits' were distinguished from symptoms on the basis that they have persisted since adolescence and there has been no exacerbation that could be regarded as an 'onset'. In Version 2, the dates of PERIODS of symptoms can be dated separately in each Section, if necessary. Trait ratings are not made.

The term 'disorder' is used as in ICD-10, "to imply the existence of a clinically recognizable set of symptoms or behaviors". Various sets of rules for recognizing such disorders are incorporated into the CATEGO computer programs, not in the SCAN text. The main sets of rules are those in the Diagnostic Criteria for Research of ICD-10 and in the DSM manuals. Any nosological system with sufficiently operationalized rules can be accommodated, perhaps with an item supplement.

Thus, the SCAN text is 'bottom-up', in the sense that it provides a means of gathering data according to the Glossary definitions, independently of the type of 'top-down' classification applied. These data can be used to provide profiles and scores of many different kinds.

TEXT CONVENTIONS IN SCAN

In the printed SCAN text a standard format is used for almost all items. Each has its own block of text, which can consist of up to five sub-blocks. The full format is illustrated by item **3.001**, 'Worrying'.

(1) The first line contains the item number, the item name in italic, and two open boxes (one for each of two possible episodes) for the entry of ratings. There are two dashed line boxes below the standard boxes. These are for the optional rating of attribution.

(2) The second component, also in italic, contains the main probe(s) for the item. In this case, there is only one question: 'Have you worried a great deal during [PERIOD]?', but there can be several.

(3) The third component contains optional probes in italic, preceded by a hyphen. In this case, five extra probes are suggested.

(4) The fourth component follows after a blank line. This is a brief reminder, of the item-definition, sometimes also a note about the rating scale.

(5) The fifth component, the rating scale, is also preceded by a blank line.

The components are also distinguished by different indentations from the left margin. These conventions are followed throughout the text of SCAN, but not all items require all five components.

Rarely, probe questions have the initial black marker but no item number, name or box. This happens above the cut-off point in Section 1 and in a few other places. The marker is there to draw attention to the need to ask the probe.

ABBREVIATIONS

Commonly used abbreviations include:

R:	Respondent.
S:	Section.
PS:	Present State.
LB:	Lifetime Before.
RE:	Representative Episode.
PY:	Past Year.
ICD-10-DCR:	International Classification of Diseases, 10th edition, Diagnostic Criteria for Research.
DSM-III-R:	Diagnostic and Statistical Manual, 3rd edition, Revised.
DSM-IV:	Diagnostic and Statistical Manual, 4th edition.

CUT-OFF POINTS

These indicate a skip to the next Section. They are shown by the words CUT OFF in the left margin, followed by => and instructions, with a continuous line below.

SKIP POINTS

These indicate movement to another item in the same section. They are shown by SKIP in the left margin, followed by => and instructions, but no line.

GENERAL POINTS ABOUT RATING SCALES I-IV AND OTHER SCALES

There are four main rating scales, placed at the beginning of the sections in which they are used.

Rating Scale I is placed immediately before Section 3 and is the main scale used in Sections 3 to 6.

Rating Scale II is placed immediately before Section 16 and is the main scale used in Sections 16 to 19.

Rating Scale III is placed at the beginning of Section 22, and is the main scale for rating Sections 22 to 25.

Rating Scale IV is placed at the beginning of Section 26, the Item Group Checklist.

The optional etiology attribution scale is placed following Scale I and Scale II, and can be used at any item with the optional etiology boxes. These boxes are located below the episode rating boxes and nave dashed instead of solid lines. The reliability or validity of etiological attributions at the item have not been systematically studied. Further investigation may be desirable in spedcific projects. Interested users should contact their training center for further information on the availability of data entry and classification algorithms using this scale.

Many symptom and behavior items have their own individual rating scales, specified within their own item blocks. It should be noted that all such items can be rated at points 0, 8 and 9, using the definitions in the four main Scales, whether or not these points are specified in the text.

There is only one universal rule: **'always rate down.'** False negatives are generally less troublesome than false positives.

0   Face sheet and sociodemographic items

0.001 - 0.020   Face Sheet

The Face Sheet provides important identifying data and other information essential to the proper running of the computer programs. It should invariably be completed carefully and checked before the data are entered. When using the laptop version, this checking process is particularly important. The choice of episodes, and the use of the non-routine option, are described in Section 1 below.

The use of the Clinical History Schedule (item **0.015**) in research studies is recommended because of its value for international co-morbidity and descriptive studies. The World Health Organization intends to compile a library of data from SCAN series. At the least it is useful to enter an independent clinical diagnosis at items **27.083 - 27.088**.

0.021 - 0.029 Sociodemographic items

These items, like those in the CHS, are optional but recommended. They are used to provide descriptive statistical profiles from series of SCAN cases. This output can be obtained at once if the laptop version of SCAN is used.

Beginning the interview

INTRODUCTION

The Section starts with the instruction that the interviewer should be well informed before starting the interview and be prepared for a number of possible contingencies. Apart from studies of general population samples it will usually possible to anticipate some of the likely problems in conducting the interview according to the routine recommendation. These include the following difficulties:

Severe language problems and cognitive impairment

Complete Section 15 for language disorders, items **21.065 - 21.099** (behavioral and history items for cognitive disorder), Sections 22-25 (more general behavior, affect and speech items), and Clinical History Schedule.

Severe behavior disturbance, R uncooperative or likely to terminate prematurely

Begin with those Sections that are most relevant to R. Keep the conversation going as far as possible and observe speech, affect and behavior (items **21.065 - 21.087**, Sections 22-25).

If necessary complete the examination in stages. All stages can be rated on one schedule if the whole is completed within a few days. Be sure to rate adequacy items.

Re-interview with PSE10 as opportunity affords. If interview is impossible, rate PS on the Item Group Checklist, and use all information available to rate Item Group Checklist for previous episode if appropriate. Complete the Clinical History Schedule.

Recent catastrophic trauma or psychosocial stressor

If SCAN cannot be completed first, complete items **13.055 - 13.128** for stress and adjustment disorders, use information from case records or informant to check the details of the event, and complete the full SCAN as soon as possible afterwards.

Prominent dissociative disorders

Complete items **2.049 - 2.074** (dissociative symptoms), obtain information from informants and case records, and complete the full SCAN.

Drug or alcohol use

If the main problem, Section 11 or 12 may be taken first, but the whole of SCAN should be completed and attributions of cause and effect rated.

Eating disorders

If the main problem, begin with Sections 8-9, then return to Section 1 and complete SCAN.

In general

Begin with Section 1, but then take Sections the respondent most wants to discuss or that are clearly predominant in the clinical picture. This will provide a more complete interview on the important topics. If the interview is likely to be incomplete, try to take sections with highly relevant items first.

DATING EPISODES AND PERIODS

Ten broad types of symptoms and signs are rated in SCAN. It has already been emphasized that the terminology used is purely descriptive. Symptoms associated with alcohol and drug use, and eating problems, form a group of 'habit disorders' that are often accompanied (whether by cause, effect or chance) by neurotic, affective or psychotic symptoms. Stress, somatoform and dissociative symptoms can be associated with any of the foregoing. Cognitive impairment can similarly produce or complicate any of the other types.

Somewhat different methods are used to choose and date periods of time that can represent clinically significant 'episodes' of each type of symptom or sign. The methods are described in detail in the Training Pack. In the SCAN text, instructions are provided in the relevant Sections of the PSE, as follows:

Cognitive impairment and decline

Rated in PSE10 Section 21. Only the Present State (PS) is rated.

Alcohol and drug use problems

Rated in PSE10 Sections 11 and 12. Two periods can be rated: Past Year, or year before key date (PY), and Lifetime Before (LB) or period from onset to PY.

Somatoform and dissociative symptoms

Rated in PSE10 Section 2. Rated for Past 2 Years (PY) for somatoform disorders.

Eating problems

Rated in PSE10 Section 9. Rated for Past Year (PY) and representative (previous) Episode (RE).

Psychotic, affective and neurotic symptoms

These types of symptom can co-present with any of the four types listed above. They are rated in PSE10 Sections 3-10, 16-20, and 22-25. Two periods can be rated: Present State (PS) and either Representative (previous) Episode (RE) **OR** Lifetime Before (LB). General instructions for rating them are provided in Section 1.

1   Introduction and overview

GENERAL POINTS ABOUT SECTION 1

If none of the special contingencies described earlier determine otherwise, and if the Special Episode List is not being used, it is recommended that the examiner routinely begin the interview with Section 1. This is because neurotic, affective and psychotic symptoms are likely to accompany any of the other types, and it is sensible to get the overall pattern of the clinical history clear, in collaboration with the respondent, before deciding where best to start.

Note the instruction that the examiner should be as fully informed as possible before beginning the interview. Points in the case records or made by informants can be used with careful discretion as extra prompts.

1.001 - 1.017   Preliminary questions on the course

Note that, at the beginning of the interview, there are several probes marked by small black squares without item numbers, names or rating boxes. It is important to cover the points indicated by these probes. The way this preliminary part of the interview is conducted is at the discretion of the examiner, using all the information at disposal to obtain a general overview of the history of clinically significant neurotic, affective or psychotic symptoms. The overall descriptive definition is 'symptoms included in Sections 3 to 10, 15 to 19, and 22 to 25 of PSE10'.

Once the presence of clinically significant periods of any of these symptom-types is decided, the interview is focused on agreeing, with the respondent, the approximate dates of the periods that will be discussed. This must be a collaborative effort, particularly if, say, two episodes out of a complex clinical history are to be rated. Both the interviewer and respondent have to be able to orient themselves correctly in order to rate them appropriately.

This review should culminate by assessing the dates of first onset of the main types of problem. It is usually most convenient to enter these as ages of first onset.

No probes are suggested to cover the 'habit' or cognitive or Section 2 symptom-types, but if they can be included in a natural way into the flow of the interview at this stage, it is wise to cover them. However, there is no need to date the time periods of these problems in this Section.

1.007 - 1.024   General points about defining and dating episodes

An episode is a period of time throughout which clinically significant symptoms persist with no symptom-free intervals lasting 3 months or more. Such an episode could last a few days or many years.

Three rating periods are recognized by the CATEGO computer program: PS, RE and LB. Although PS primarily refers to the clinical state of the subject for the past month, PS is also used to refer to a representative part of a much longer episode, which has not yet clearly remitted. It is important to keep in mind these two subtly different meanings and uses of the PS. RE is a previous episode characterized chiefly by one of the three types of symptom. LB is a period containing more than one episode. All three can be rated by using either PSE10 or IGC.

Dates are determined by clinical judgement. Detailed probes are not laid down, since the proceedings must be conducted according to the unique clinical history of each respondent and in the interest of creating a relationship between examiner and respondent that will provide a solid basis of trust on which to build the interview. The information needed is complex, private, confidential and difficult for the respondent to describe in terms that are sufficiently quantifiable to make it comparable with the descriptions provided by other people. The object of the SCAN interview is to create the conditions in which this transfer of communication can nevertheless take place.

PRESENT STATE (PS)

PS represents the clinical state present during the month before the date of examination. As was the case with PSE9, the term 'month' should be understood as notional or approximate; it could be extended up to 6 weeks or so, depending on the interviewer's clinical judgement. The episode need not have begun during the month. In other words, the PS also may be part of a much longer 'present episode' (PE), with onset years earlier. In other words, PS either fully constitutes, or is the most recent part of, a PE. The onset of the PE is defined by at least 3 months without clinically significant symptoms. The length in months of this episode is entered at item **1.006**. This allows the calculation of the date of onset of the episode.

If the Present State is part of a continuous episode that has lasted longer than a month, with many characteristic symptoms still present but with a peak somewhat more than the 'notional month' ago, it is permissible to extend the period a little in order to accommodate the most characteristic symptoms within the PS. The most common occasion is likely to be when a patient has been admitted to hospital and has recovered to some extent before the interview. In longer chronic illness, if the PE extends back in time considerably further and some significant symptoms manifest then are no longer present, these could be rated using RE or LB. The number of days covered by the PS is recorded at item **1.008**, so that it is clear how comparable the results are with those of others in the series. When SCAN is used to structure the interview with people who do not have significant clinical symptoms at examination, the PSE Part One should be completed for the previous month, consisting of all the above-cut-off items and the Screen (Check-PSE). This occurs most frequently:

(a) In a population or general practice survey, where many respondents will not be in episode as defined above;

(b) In clinical situations where acute episodes are infrequent, for example in follow up clinics, long-stay wards, day centers or hostels;

(c) When the disorder is only minor or takes the form of negative symptoms, and the most characteristic clinical pictures have occurred in previous episodes.

(d) When the Respondent has long-term and clinically significant problems on examination that have lasted perhaps for years, but cannot be split up into episodes because fluctuations are not sufficiently marked. Examples might include very long-term dysthymic or somatoform disorders, and personality disorders with occasional minor symptoms. In such cases, the whole course of the condition constitutes one episode as defined in SCAN. Because significant symptoms are present during the month before examination, no symptom-free period lasting 3+ months is included, and there are no significant symptoms during the 3 months before onset, PS is the appropriate period to rate. If it lasts throughout the whole clinical course, from early adolescence, it is a form of 'lifetime ever'. However, it does not need a special designation since PS represents the whole course.

If the time of symptom onset varies according to the type of symptom, a separate date of onset can be recorded in each Section of PSE-10. PS can be rated in the Item Group Checklist, from case records or an informant, if the Respondent is unwilling or unable to supply information.

PREVIOUS EPISODE

A previous episode is any period of clinically significant symptoms occurring with a 3 month or greater interval without significant symptoms before the PS, and similarly separated from any other episode by at least a 3 month clear interval. One exception to this might be in the not uncommon clinical situation with long term, continuous chronic illness where there is no 3 month period without significant symptoms. When important symptoms that are not present now existed too far back in time to reasonably be included in the PS, they can be rated using the previous episode option. Two kinds are conventionally distinguished: RE and LB.

REPRESENTATIVE EPISODE (RE)

If there has been one particular episode before PS which, alone or in combination with PS, provides an adequate coverage of the significant clinical symptomatology for diagnostic purposes, it is dated and designated a Representative Episode (RE). It should be chosen by consultation with R. A notional month at the peak of the disorder will be most informative. RE will usually be used in association with PS. It can also be rated using the Item Group Checklist, if the Respondent is unable or unwilling to provide details and if good records and/or a good informant are available. Once RE is chosen, the dates are entered at item **1.009**.

Three common uses for RE are:

(a) If the Respondent is in episode (PS) at the time of interview, and RE contains symptoms of similar type but with a more characteristic symptom profile, it will often be useful to rate both episodes: PS + RE.

(b) If PS and one particular RE contain different clinical pictures (for example, manic and depressive symptoms), the two sets of ratings will be processed separately.

(c) If R is not in episode at the time of interview (as confirmed by the Check-PS), RE is the chief source of information about a single past episode.

LIFETIME BEFORE (LB)

LB is dated from the first onset of disorder to the beginning of the period covered in PS. PS+LB therefore constitute another form of 'lifetime ever'. LB is mainly used when there have been several previous episodes, whether discrete or merging into each other, that contain different types of symptom - e.g. psychotic, affective and neurotic - with the possibility of several diagnoses. It may then be necessary (depending on the nature of the Present State) to choose different peak periods for two episodes with different types of symptom but to rate them as though they were sub-episodes of one extended episode. The dates of episodes rated in LB are rated under the relevant symptom type at items **1.010** to **1.013**.

The routine CATEGO program processes the information as part of one episode but, if sub-episodes are specified by symptom type and date, the relevant parts of the data can be identified for each separately. It should be emphasized that identifying the symptom type of an episode does not compromise the independence of the classification since the CATEGO program does not take this information into account when categorizing. It is, in any case, symptomatic, not diagnostic. Symptom scores and Item Group profiles, however, can only be provided for the whole of LB.

It is also possible to record the date of previous Episodes separately in each Section.

1.014 - 1.017   Age of first onset of symptom types

1.018   Quality of remissions between episodes

This item should be rated using all the information at disposal. If the respondent has had more than one episode of depression (Section 6) or of elation (Section 10), the dating of previous episodes should be recorded in those Sections (**6.038 - 6.043** and **10.022 - 10.027**) taking account of the rating of item **1.018**.

1.019 - 1.024   Special episode list (Option)

Rating LB does not provide a full PSE profile for each type of disorder rated during the overall period. For projects that require this degree of detail, an 'episode list' should be completed instead of PS and LB. This allows the specification of up to six dated episodes (or periods), each of which can be rated using the full PSE10, or IGC, or some of either. Each episode is processed separately and the Project Director would be responsible for putting the results together. For some very detailed research projects it may be useful to complete both the routine and the non-routine options for each member of the series.

1.025 - 1.036   Medication

This list of items is included in order to record the use of various kinds of medication at the time of interview and the effect this has had on symptoms (item **1.035**) and on the interview itself (item **1.036**).

1.037 - 1.042   Psychosocial treatments

This list performs a similar purpose to the previous list (i.e. medication).

1.043 - 1.052   Other aspects of clinical history

These items provide an additional view of the clinical history that can be used in conjunction with co-morbidity studies to compare symptom, Item Group or category profiles.

Rating scales in Part One

GENERAL POINTS

The main rating scale in Sections 3-6 is Scale I. The rating points are specified in the SCAN text, at the beginning of Section 3, and elaborated on the next page of the Glossary.

However, many items (particularly in other sections of Part One) have their own individual rating scales, which are specified within their item blocks. It should be noted that all symptom items can be rated at points 0, and 5-9, using the definitions given in Scale I, whether or not these points are specified in the text.

For making etiological attributions, many items have boxes with dashed line below the episode rating boxes. These are optional ratings that are not required, but which may be useful for research purposes, and in certain clinical situations. The purpose is to separate the ratings of phenomenology from any ratable etiological factors for example Parkinson's disease, or the effects of alcohol or other drugs. The etiology scale should be used to code any attribution of etiology.

RATING SEVERITY

The severity of a symptom can be assessed in terms of duration, persistence, degree of interference with other mental functions, distress, impairment of everyday activities, effect on other people, and contact with services of various kinds. In SCAN, the approach is to measure clinical severity by the duration and frequency of the symptom and the degree of interference with mental functions (intensity). Social and occupational performance, other people's reactions, and help-seeking behavior (all of which can be influenced by many other factors), are assessed separately.

Somewhere between the two lies the respondent's own reaction, but this may be stoical or distressed according to temperament and circumstances, and is therefore also regarded as adding a degree of ambiguity to the rating. Distress is only mentioned in items which use criteria from a rule-based system that requires it to be present.

These points hold good for ratings throughout SCAN and, in particular, for the four main Rating Scales.

RATING SCALE I

Many items in Sections 3-6 are rated on this standard 4-point scale (0-3). The factors chiefly involved are intensity (intrusiveness and extent of interference with mental functions) and frequency of the symptoms. The standard definitions are suitable for a period of about 4 to 6 weeks. This is the period of the 'Present State', from which the PSE originally derived its name.

In longer episodes, it is often possible to select (with R) a period of equivalent length during which most of the symptoms characteristic of the episode were present (a 'representative month').

When rating a period longer than a month it may be difficult to specify the proportion of time during which a symptom has been present.

In such cases, rate mainly on clinical intensity rather than duration. Frequency can still, however, be used as appropriate.

Do not be too pedantic when asking about each symptom. It is usually sufficient to establish an overall frequency and intensity for a group of symptoms and then to establish any variation in particular items.

0. This is a positive rating of absence. It does not mean 'not known' or 'uncertain whether present or not'. It can only be used if sufficient information is available to establish its accuracy.

1. This is a positive rating of presence, but presence of such a minor degree that it is not appropriate for use in classification. Like (0), it does not mean 'not known' or 'uncertain'. Ratings of (1) count in scores, which in turn influence the level allocated on the Index of Definition.

2. This rating means that the item is present at a level sufficient to use in classification. For this purpose it is equivalent to 3, but it contributes less to scores. In general, it is used when symptoms are of moderate severity during most of the period being assessed.

3. A rating of (3) is similar to (2) except that the symptom is present in severe form for most of the period under review.

5. The presence of psychotic symptoms can make the rating of Part One items very difficult, because of problems in interpreting the meaning of what R says, or because the symptoms (for example, anxiety or a phobia about leaving one's house) may themselves be based in psychotic experiences. The rating should only be made when there is genuine doubt about the nature of the symptom or the balance is in favor of the symptom being psychotic.

8. If, after an adequate examination, the interviewer is still not sure whether a symptom is present (rated 1-3) or absent (rated 0), the rating is (8). This is the only circumstance in which (8) is used. It should not be used to indicate a mild form of the symptom.

9. This rating is only used if the information needed to rate an item is incomplete in some respect, for example because of language or cognitive disorder, or lack of cooperation, or because the interviewer forgot to probe sufficiently deeply. It is distinguished from (8) because the examination was not, for whatever reason, carried out adequately.

In the SCAN text, an instruction to 'use Scale I' simply means that it is not necessary to point out any individual rating characteristics for that item. Any point on Scale I can be selected, according to clinical judgement.

OPTIONAL RATINGS OF ITEM-SPECIFIC ATTRIBUTIONS OF CAUSES AND TRAIT RATINGS

The following optional ratings should only be made by investigators planning to study their validity. The reliability of making these ratings should be established. They represent a more detailed way of recording ratings of attribution of organic cause throughout the SCAN. There is also an opportunity to make a trait rating of individual items (i.e. a rating of "7" on rating SCALE I of SCAN version 1). Users should contact their training center of up to date information of their employment in SCAN algorithms.

SCAN users and raters with qualification and practice experience in medicine and clinical pharmacology, studying patients following appropriate, extensive, physical and laboratory investigation way wish to rate judgements of definite attributions of cause at an item level. Only attributions that can be positively rated should be entered. For each period first rate the item using the appropriate SCAN rating scale (I-IV), in the standard scoring boxes, and then the nature of the attribution in the dashed boxes below the standard boxes, using the scale provided. Up to two periods can be rated. Note that the conventional use of 0,8, and 9 does not apply and these scores have specific meaning. The items themselves already should have been rated purely on the basis of certainty, presence, and severity.

ATTRIBUTIONAL RATING SCALE (Optional)

Use the Attributional Rating Scale to rate the nature of influence on symptom presence or severity.

1 Alcohol
2 Other psychoactive substance
3 Effects of somatic psychiatric treatments (electroconvulsive therapy, antidepressant medication, neuroleptics, etc)
4 Known primary intracranial process (Alzheimer's disease, Huntington's disease, Parkinson's disease, tumor, stroke, etc.)
5 Non-psychiatric medication, toxins
6 Other medication condition 1 (specify at Section 13 and/or Section 20)
7 Other medication condition 2 (specify at Section 13 and/or Section 20)
8 Other medication condition 3 (specify at Section 13 and/or Section 20)
9 Trait. Essentially lifelong characteristic of R.

2 Physical health, somatoform and dissociative disorders

GENERAL POINTS ABOUT SOMATOFORM SYMPTOMS

The somatoform symptoms considered in this Section require an assurance that 'no adequate physical explanation has been found'. This does not imply that a full explanation in physical terms is impossible, since knowledge is not that far advanced. The same caveat applies to all the symptoms and behavioral signs that are rated in SCAN.

The somatoform subsection begins with items (**2.001 - 2.009**) concerned with general physical health and well-being. This provides enough information to establish whether somatoform or dissociative symptoms (**2.010 - 2.048**, and **2.049 - 2.074**) are present. If the examiner considers that there is, or probably is, a physical explanation for all the clinically significant symptoms described by R, skip out of the Section altogether. The cut-off point is always passed if there is any doubt. An optional checklist provides a comprehensive list of somatoform symptoms (**2.080 - 2.135**), including those required for DSM somatization disorder. This can supplement the briefer grouped list (**2.010 - 2.035**), for ICD-10 criteria in the text.

The period rated is usually the past year but provision is made for rating age of onset of the first and present episodes. If an earlier episode is needed for research purposes, the Special Episodes List (see items **0.016** and **1.019 - 1.024**) can be used.

It is particularly important to use all the information at disposal when rating Section 2 items, including informants, case records and the results of clinical investigations.

Most items are rated 0 or 1; the latter meaning that a clinically significant proportion of the symptoms cannot fully be explained by physical illness. If investigations are incomplete or services are inadequate to provide a proper workup, the rating should be cautious; full use should be made of 'not known' (8). If some symptoms are 'somatoform' while a physical explanation is probably justifiable in the case of some others, the latter should be rated 9 (not applicable) or 8 (uncertain).

2.001 Physical fitness, past month

This item is concerned with the Respondent's own view of his or her own physical health status; i.e. not only with the presence or absence of disease or disability but also with general physical well-being. Respondents will use their own terms to describe health status. The rating should reflect this personal assessment rather than interviewer's interpretation of it. A rating of 1 must be based on a positive statement of physical well-being. Reasonably well (rated 2) corresponds to 'all right'; not positive, not negative. A rating of 3 ('fair') implies less than average fitness. Such a statement should be elucidated to inform subsequent questioning. It may, for example, indicate physical disorder, somatoform or dissociative or affective disorder, or a lifelong tendency (trait) to take a somewhat gloomy view of things. These questions are raised later in the interview. Any statement implying a seriously poor state of health, is rated 4.

A feeling of positive fitness can be rated 1 in the presence of actual disease or disability if that is what R feels.

The scale is ordered in this way (1-4) to correspond with the general principle used elsewhere in the SCAN text, that greater disability or pathology has a higher score. Thus 0 is not used, because, as the default rating for all items (except some in Section 20), it would automatically indicate high positive fitness if left blank.

2.002 Length of unfitness

If item **2.001** is rated 3 or 4, specify the length of time in years and months that the unfitness has been present.

2.003 Change in weight, past year

Weight loss or gain may be associated with many mental and physical disorders. This item is purely descriptive; a useful probe to orient subsequent questioning. Two kilograms (5 lbs in the UK) within a brief period (up to six weeks) is taken as the arbitrary threshold between major and minor change. More precise information is coded at items **8.001 - 8.008**. Clearly described change in weight during the current episode qualifies for a positive rating, even if weight has returned to normal (e.g. as a result of treatment). Weight loss due to controlled dieting is included.

If weight loss is deliberate and induced by a fear of fatness or there are deviant eating attitudes, the interviewer should consider continuing with Section 9 on eating disorders.

If R is unsure, or unused to measures of weight, an approximate scale can be used, e.g.: 0, no change; 1, minor change; 2, major loss; 3, major gain; 4, major fluctuation in weight.

2.004 - 2.006 Physical illnesses or disabilities, past year

These items refer to medical problems of a physical nature including illnesses, injuries and disabilities. Take into account all the information available including the results of recent investigations and examinations. It will sometimes be possible to accept the diagnosis that R gives, when backed by a convincing description, but always use 8 if there is doubt. Any medically diagnosed condition should be coded in **2.005** and **2.006**, according to ICD-10. If no significant illness or disability is present leave **2.005** and **2.006** blank. An entry should only be made if **2.044** is coded 2; not including any indefinite or medically unexplained disorder. For instance stomach ache without good evidence of gastric disease, should not be entered simply because R states, for example, "I think I have a gastric ulcer". A rating of 1 does not mean that there is no physical disease, only that the information has not established one and further enquiry is necessary.

2.007 Premenstrual Symptoms

This item must be rated on the basis of the presence of any one of eight symptoms specified in the schedule which emerge a few days before menstruation and cease immediately the period begins. Ideally such a rating should be based on a diary covering at least two cycles and having specific reference to the key symptoms. If this is not available, the rating must be made on a careful history of symptoms over several cycles. The symptoms must be related in the manner described to almost all recent cycles. The effects of a positive response set on the part of the subject, together with leading questions from the interviewer, should be kept in mind. (This is, of course, a general principle for interviewing.) The period rated is, in general, the past year.

The symptoms may also occur after hysterectomy although menstruation is absent, because of central (hypothalamic) hormonal regulation.

Differentiation from other symptoms:

Distinguish dysmenorrhea (painful menses) where the symptoms are associated only with the duration of the menses. Premenstrual aggravation or exacerbation of any existing mental disorder such as anxiety disorders or depressive disorders should not count since they do not remit after the onset of the menses. However, if R experiences characteristic symptoms which are markedly different from those of the co-existing disorder, the item may be rated positively.

2.008 Limitation of activities or well-being

Restriction of daily life activities because of medical problems rated present in items **2.001 - 2.007**. Please note that any limitation or deficit caused by a medical disorder might well be overcome by the development of compensating skills or the use of medical aids or prostheses. The interviewer should rate the respondent's assessment of any limitation.

2.009 Satisfaction with the advice/care provided

This item is part of the screen for somatoform and dissociative disorders. If the respondent is satisfied with the investigations carried out and the explanations offered, and if it is clear that any physical symptoms present can be explained by physical disease or disability, skip to Section 3.

It may sometimes be useful to take other sections first, e.g. Section 4 if there is marked anxiety or Section 6-8 if there is marked depression, returning to Section 2 if a somatoform condition requires further exploration.

CUT-OFF POINT

Always continue beyond the cut-off point if there is any doubt as to whether physical health problems have a clearly physical origin. Begin the further exploration with a general probe, then ask a set of questions concerning R's contacts with expert practitioners. In countries where expert opinion is difficult to obtain the following ratings must be particularly circumspect. Case records and information from people who know R should be taken into account.

2.010 - 2.035   List of grouped somatoform symptoms

2.080 - 2.135   Extended list of somatoform symptoms

These two lists cover items related to autonomic dysfunctions, which can be manifested in many and varying ways. To rate a symptom as present, establish that it is not fully explained by any detectable organic pathology or demonstrated cause; and that it has given rise to multiple consultations with doctors (local healers, etc.), self-medication and/or change of life-style. Use the list of probes on page xx of the SCAN text, in addition to information from case records and knowledgeable informants, to establish the extent to which the problems have been investigated.

Because each symptom can be described in terms that are highly culture specific, neither list can be exhaustive. There are sufficient items to cover contingencies. A clinical decision has to be made on the basis of expert local knowledge as to which item represents the complaint most closely. For research purposes, it would be important to record the terms used by respondents to describe their problems.

Each item in the first list, if affirmed, can be assessed using the listed probes concerning contacts with experts. This will form a context in which the rest of the Section 2 interview will be carried out. The items allow ratings of groups of similar symptoms.

The usual PSE rule 'if in doubt rate down' should not be applied to somatoform symptoms themselves. Respondents should be encouraged to be forthcoming about their complaints. However, this does not alter the rule that these complaints must not be caused by detectable physical pathology.

If more specific detail is required, e.g. for DSM disorders, or for research purposes, or because of the likelihood of the local occurrence of particular patterns of symptoms, the list at **2.080 - 2.135** provides extended coverage.

Brief descriptions of items **2.010- 2.035** are provided below, including the symptoms covered by each.

2.010   Shortness of breath when not exercising

Cannot breathe easily; smothering or choking feeling; difficulty in breathing; present when not making much effort.

2.011 **Chest or heart pain, discomfort, burning**

Aches, pains, pressure, burning, stinging feelings in the chest or over the heart.

2.012 **Vomiting, regurgitation**

Vomiting, belching, regurgitation of food.

2.013 **Difficulty with swallowing**

Feeling a lump in the throat ('globus hystericus').

2.014 **Stomach or bowel pain, wind, indigestion**

Abdominal pain, cramps due to wind, bowel spasms, constipation. Intolerance to several kinds of food should also be rated here. Rate bad taste in mouth at **2.034** and loose bowels at **2.035**.

2.015 **Problems with passing water, frequency**

Pain or burning sensation during urination, difficulty, retention, frequency of passing water, sense of urgency, or any similar urinary complaint.

2.016 **Pain in arms or limbs, joints hands or feet**

Aches or pains in muscles, limbs, joints and extremities, including pains 'wandering' round different parts of the body.

2.017 **Headache**

It covers headaches only.

2.018 **Loss of memory**

Loss of memory for certain (often stressful) events, covering a period of hours or more. The loss does not include anaesthesia for operations or during convulsions or fainting, or following head injury.

2.019 **Any problem with sight, hearing or speech**

This symptom group includes blindness in one or both eyes and other problems with vision (excluding blurring due to lack of proper glasses, or double vision); loss of hearing, ringing or buzzing in the ears or in the head; loss of voice; loss of speech and other problems that relate to voice, pronunciation, etc.

2.020   Convulsions, trances, faints, dizziness

This symptom group covers any sort of loss or alteration of consciousness, including light-headedness, near-fainting, trances, catalepsy, fainting, passing out, convulsions, fits, spells of unconsciousness.

2.021   Problems with movement, paralysis

This group covers muscular weakness (either periodic or unremitting). problems in lifting, inability to stand up or to walk; or inability to move any part of the body.

2.022   Numbness, loss of sensation, tingling

This symptom group covers loss of feeling in any part of the body (numbness, anaesthesia) or different sensations such as tingling (slight stinging sensation/pins and needles), crawling or creeping impressions as well as feelings of heaviness or lightness anywhere in the body.

2.023   Genital problems, pain, discomfort, discharge

Complaints such as genital discharge (e.g. loss of semen in urine); genital discomfort, burning sensations, pain during intercourse, irregular menstruations, excessive menstrual bleeding, excessive pain with menstruation, impotence, lack of sexual feeling are grouped together under this heading. Rate unusual or copious vaginal discharge at **2.033**.

2.024   Blotchy or discolored skin

Changes in skin color especially in patches.

2.025 - 2.028   Autonomic symptoms

Autonomic symptoms are specified as being particularly likely to be associated with somatoform disorders. They must have the general somatoform characteristics but they are otherwise identical with items **4.005** (**2.025**, palpitations), **4.013** (**2.026** or **2.028**, hot or cold sweats or flushes), and **4.009** (**2.027**, dry mouth not due to medication).

2.029   Churning or discomfort in stomach

This refers to constant or periodic unpleasant feelings in the stomach, an upset stomach. Foods that make the subject ill should be rated in **2.014**.

2.030   Other Pains

Aches and pains not included in items **2.011, 2.014, 2.015, 2.016, or 2.017.** (chest pain, abdominal pain, dysuria, pain in joints or extremities, headache). It covers back pain and aches or pains in any other site of the body. e.g. pain behind the neck, pain in rectum etc.

2.031   Other symptoms

This category covers symptoms not included in the preceding items.

2.032   Nausea

Feeling of disgust, revulsion, sensation that precedes vomiting.

2.033   Unusual or copious vaginal discharge

Passing of fluid, usually whitish in color and in small amounts from vagina. The amount of discharge is variable: Respondents who report this symptom often attribute their other bodily complaints to vaginal discharge.

2.034   Bad taste in mouth, excessively coated tongue

This symptom may be reported along with other gastro-intestinal symptoms such as belching, regurgitation of food, intolerance for several kinds of food or abdominal cramps but should be rated separately here.

2.035   Frequent loose bowels or fluid discharge from anus

Complaints of fluid discharge from anus, frequent or loose bowels or diarrhoea.

2.036   Length of distress due to preoccupation

This item refers to any symptoms rated present at **2.010 - 2.035**, which distress the Respondent by their persistence, although no explanation for them has been provided. Enter the number of months that the symptoms have been present.

2.037   Variability of somatoform symptoms

Somatoform symptoms tend to be multiple but are not necessarily present together at one time. Rate the frequency of variation.

2.038 Hypochondriacal preoccupation

The symptom has the characteristics of worrying (see **3.001**) but is also distinguished:

(i) By an intense preoccupation with apparently normal sensations or physical signs or appearances, which are interpreted in terms of no more than one or two serious physical illnesses;

(ii) By persistence of the preoccupation in spite of adequate and repeated investigation, and expert advice that it is groundless.

Although there are often brief periods of relief immediately following such reassurance, and the degree of conviction varies (rating of 1), the round of painful and distressing worry returns. Moderate to severe social disablement often accompanies the symptom.

Although the preoccupation may reach the force of a conviction from time to time it is more an inability to put the possibility of disease out of mind when interpreting normal sensations and signs.

Differentiation from other symptoms:

If there is true conviction of the presence of a nonexistent disease, rate at item **2.039** (repeated at **19.028** and, if in context of depressed mood, at **19.027**). Somatic hallucinations and delusional elaboration are rated at **17.028** and **17.029**.

Phobias of contracting disease (**4.044**), or of medical situations (**4.043**), should be distinguished if they lack the two characteristics specified above.

Obsessional preoccupation with the possibility of harm from contamination or infection (**5.004**), must have the characteristic resistance against subjective compulsion.

The differentiation from phobias and obsessions can be difficult. If criteria for more than one symptom are satisfied, each should be rated on its merits. One does not exclude the others.

2.039 Hypochondriacal conviction

When hypochondriacal preoccupation is most severe it takes the form of a fixed delusion that disease is present even when no abnormality is found in repeated examinations. Respondents are convinced that one (or perhaps two) diseases account for the symptoms and are not satisfied with the way that medical experts have handled the case or with the conclusions and explanations offered. They may contact one doctor (or other healer) after another and accept many treatments but totally reject assurances that there is no adequate physical cause for the symptoms, except for short periods following or during medical investigations or interventions. This item is repeated at **19.028**.

Differentiation from other symptoms:

Differentiation from phobias and obsessions should not be difficult. If it is difficult to be sure of the presence of delusional conviction, rate as item **2.038**.

2.040   Excessive and distressing fatigue [physical exercise]

Unwarranted fatiguability after even minor physical exertion. The emphasis is on feelings of bodily or physical weakness and exhaustion after only minimal effort, accompanied by a feeling of muscular aches and pains. Respondents experience the tiredness as unpleasant and distressing.

Differentiation from other symptoms:

Tiredness at the end of a hard day of physical work (rate 0), or due to the after-effect of influenza, would not count. The level of increase in fatiguability should be assessed against relevant previous experience, such as walking a familiar distance, climbing stairs, etc. Differentiate from item **3.007**, which is not necessarily related to physical exercise.

A clinical decision should be made when the disorder has been attributed by experts to a viral aetiology. Rate 9 if this is accepted and specify at item **2.078**.

2.041   Excessive and distressing fatigue [mental exercise]

The main feature is excessive mental fatigue following even minor mental exercise. This is typically described as an unpleasant intrusion of distracting associations or recollections, difficulty in concentrating, focusing and sustaining attention, and generally inefficient thinking. The condition is usually associated with decreased efficiency in coping with daily tasks.

Differentiation from other symptoms:

Tiredness at the end of a hard day's mental work (rate 0), or due to the after-effect of influenza (rate 9), would not count. The level of increase should be assessed against relevant previous experience, such as reading a book, doing calculations, etc. Differentiate from item **3.007**, which is not necessarily related to mental exercise.

2.042   Inability to recover normally from fatigue

Inability to restore mental and physical energy after excessive fatigue following even minor exercise. This is a prolongation, lasting days or longer, of the symptom rated at items **2.040** and **2.041**. The sense of tiredness is usually accompanied by feelings of muscular aches and pains, and the Respondent is unable voluntarily to overcome it. A main feature is inability to relax fully. Differentiate from normal sleepiness and from item **3.007**, which is not necessarily related to exercise. Rate 0 if R is able to recover normally from fatigue.

2.043 - 2.048   Preoccupation with symptoms within a bodily system

A marked preoccupation with groups of somatic symptoms that are all related to one particular bodily system or organ (usually one largely under autonomic control), thus partly mimicking a physical disorder of that system or organ. The symptoms are based on signs of autonomic arousal of the system.

2.043   Heart and cardiovascular:

Chest pains or discomfort in and around the precordium; palpitations.

2.044   Oesophagus and stomach:

Dry mouth, epigastric discomfort or 'butterflies' or churning in the stomach, aerophagy, belching, feeling of being bloated, distended or heavy, intolerance to several kinds of foods.

2.045   Lower gastro-intestinal tract:

Reported increase in frequency of bowel movements.

2.046   Respiratory system:

Dyspnea or hyperventilation.

2.047   Urogenital system:

Increased frequency of micturition or dysuria.

2.048   Other psychosomatic problem

2.049   Pain syndrome associated with stress

The predominant complaint is a persistent and distressing pain that cannot be explained by a physical disorder, occurring in association with emotional conflict or psychosocial problems. The 'stress' caused by these emotional or psychosocial problems should be sufficient to allow the conclusion that they are the main causative factors.

Pain presumed to be of psychogenic origin occurring during the course of depressive disorders or schizophrenia should not be included.

2.050   Pain syndrome not associated with stress

As **2.049**, but not associated with stress.

2.051   Elaboration of physical symptoms

These are symptoms originally caused by, or associated with, some physical disorder, which are exaggerated or prolonged by psychological factors such as compensation, fear of death, or hope for more successful treatment. (This item is repeated at **27.069** because of the need for information from other sources.)

Differentiation from other symptoms:

The main difference is from malingering. A clinical judgement has to be made in the light of all the evidence as to whether the motivation is or is not conscious. See the general comments under Dissociative Symptoms, below.

2.052   Factitious disorder

A persistent pattern of intentional production or feigning of symptoms and/or self-infliction of wounds in order to produce symptoms in the absence of a confirmed physical or mental disorder. (This item is repeated at **27.068** because of the need for information from other sources.)

Includes Munchausen's syndrome. A recent description of such a condition is as follows: *"A 21 year old man presented in casualty saying that he had taken 10 paracetamol tablets, 45 phenytoin tablets, a lot of alcohol and had injected an unknown substance. On admission to a medical ward he added that he had swallowed two razor blades and four nails. Radiography showed this to be so. Shortly afterwards he swallowed a ward thermometer, which was shown to be broken and the mercury spilled at re-X-ray. During the night he claimed to hear voices instructing him, was noisy, abusive, uncooperative, and assaulted a female nurse."* He had a fresh midline abdominal scar probably resulting from laparotomy following a similar previous episode. He said it had been for a bleeding ulcer but would not name the hospital. All the relatives' addresses he gave proved false.

Differentiation from other symptoms:

If evidence can be found for a conscious external motivation (such as financial compensations, escape from danger, or more medical care) the appropriate code is for malingering (Z76.5 in ICD-10).

DISSOCIATIVE SYMPTOMS

GENERAL POINTS ABOUT DISSOCIATIVE SYMPTOMS

Dissociative symptoms are all characterized by a partial or complete disconnection between memories of the past, awareness of identity and of immediate sensations, and control of bodily movements. Conscious control over which memories and sensations can be selected for immediate attention, and what movements can be carried out, is impaired, although varying in degree from day to day and even from hour to hour. The severity of impairment is often difficult to determine clinically.

The terms 'hysteria' and 'conversion' are avoided in ICD-10, and dissociative symptoms are presumed to be 'psychogenic' in origin, because closely associated with traumatic events, intolerable or insoluble problems, or disturbed relationships. No particular theory of the mechanisms underlying dissociation is assumed for purposes of this Glossary but secondary gain is a suggestive feature.

People with dissociative symptoms often deny problems that are obvious to others. An informant is then essential for proper rating.

See also items **17.020**, dissociative hallucinations, and **19.052 - 19.029**, which constitute the Checklist for Induced Psychosis.

For a definite rating the following features must be present:

1. The clinical characteristics specified at each item.
2. Some evidence of psychological causation - e.g. convincing temporal association with stressful events, relationship or other problems or needs - often denied by the respondent. This requires a clinical judgement, usually based also on information from another informant.
3. The presence of any relevant disorder of the central or peripheral nervous system should be specified at items **2.077** and **2.078**. If this fully explains the symptom, rate 9.
4. Positive ratings should never be made if the appropriate physical investigations have not been carried out. Rate 8 in this case.

Differentiation from other symptoms:

Depersonalization and derealization are not associated with loss of conscious control over access to sensations, memories or movements, and only limited aspects of personal identity are affected. In depersonalization, there may be a loss of the sense of self, but the people affected know who they are.

2.053   Dissociative amnesia

The main feature is loss of memory, usually of important recent events, not due to organic mental disorder and too great to be explained by ordinary forgetfulness or fatigue. There is no integration of present experiences with memories of the past. The amnesia is presumed to be of psychogenic origin and is usually partial and selective. The main problem is not in the registration or retention of the memory, but in the recall of facts usually associated with insoluble or unacceptable interpersonal problems, or traumatic events such as accidents or unexpected bereavements. The loss of memory may be an expression of emotional needs or failure of effective coping mechanisms.

Differentiation from other symptoms:

There should be no evidence of a physical disorder that can explain the symptoms that characterize the disorder. Amnesia induced by alcohol or drugs, or by postictal amnesia in epilepsy, should not be included here. Similarly subjective complaints of loss of memory (difficulty in recollection of important facts and events) experienced in depressive disorders should be distinguished.

2.054　Amnesia centered round recent stress

As item **2.053** convincingly associated in time with traumatic events, disturbed social relationships or insoluble problems.

2.055　Fugue associated with stress

Apparently purposeful travel beyond the usual everyday range in an amnesic state. The subject's behavior during the fugue may appear completely normal to independent observers. However, respondents display a complete dissociative amnesia about the events during that period. There should be evidence for psychological causation in the form of convincing associations in time with stressful events, problems or needs.

2.056　Dissociative stupor

A condition of psychogenic origin in which there is a profound diminution or absence of voluntary movement and normal responsiveness to external stimuli such as light, noise and touch. The muscle tone is maintained together with normal breathing and limited coordinated eye movements. There should be positive evidence of psychogenic causation in the form of recent stressful events or problems and a clear-cut absence of evidence for a physical cause.

Differentiation from other symptoms:

This condition should be distinguished from catatonia (items **21.021 - 21.030**) and stupor (items **20.065, 20.066** and **21.006**).

2.057　Trance

A temporary loss of the sense of personal identity and full awareness of the surroundings or limitation of movements, postures, and speech to repetition of a small repertoire.

2.058　Possession experience

A feeling that the individual has been taken over, without wishing it, by a spirit, power, deity or other person. Distinguish from alienation experiences as described in Section 18.

2.059   Possession experience combined with trance

Definitions as in **2.057** and **2.058**.

2.060   Dissociative convulsions

Convulsions which may mimic epileptic seizures in which whole or parts of the body shakes. However, these are usually longer in duration, and tongue-biting, bruising due to falling, incontinence of urine are rare. There is not a true loss of consciousness, but a state of trance or dissociative stupor. A positive rating should not be made without full neurological investigation.

2.061   Association of 2.055 - 2.060 with stress

All dissociative disorders are presumed to be of psychogenic origin. Onset is convincingly associated in time with a traumatic life event, with intolerable or insoluble problems, or with disturbed interpersonal relationships, which R may not acknowledge or be aware of. Loss of consciousness or any other bodily function may be a sign of emotional need or conflict. A disinterested informant is usually necessary.

Differentiation from other symptoms:

There should be no evidence of a physical disorder that can explain the symptoms that characterize the disorder (but physical disorders may be present that give rise to other symptoms).

2.062   Dissociative sensory loss or anaesthesia

There is a declared sensory loss on the skin which often has boundaries that do not fit into any neurological deficit. These may be associated with different sensations like tingling or other paraesthesias. There may be differential loss between the sensory modalities (touch, pain, heat, vibration, etc.) which cannot be due to a neurological problem.

This item also covers the partial or complete loss of vision, hearing or smell which is of psychogenic origin.

2.063   Association of 2.063 with stress

See **2.061**.

2.064   Dissociative disorder of voluntary movement

The loss of ability to move the whole or a part of body or limbs. This item also includes speech. These may mimic any neurological deficit such as astasia abasia, akinesia, apraxia, aphonia, dysarthria, dyskinesia, paraparesis or paralysis.

2.065   Association of 2.065 with stress

See **2.061.**

2.066 - 2.069   Multiple personality

The existence of two or more distinct personalities within the individual, only one being evident at a time. Each personality has its own memories, preferences and behavior patterns, and at some time (and recurrently) takes full control of the individual's behavior. There is inability to recall important personal information which is too intensive to be explained by ordinary forgetfulness. The condition is of psychogenic origin. The personalities are not merely different facets of a single personality disorder but are distinct coherent identities, each with an enduring pattern of perceiving, relating and thinking.

2.070   Other dissociative states

This is a residual category to include transient amnesic or trance states of adolescence, Ganser's syndrome, poorly differentiated multiple personality, psychogenic confusion and twilight states.

2.071 - 2.074   Ages of onset

These may be approximate but if there are somatoform or dissociative symptoms it is more useful to enter an estimated age (say, within 5 years) than to leave the boxes blank. If any estimate could be grossly wrong, enter 88.

2.075   Dates of PERIOD of Section 2 symptoms

2.076   Interference with activities due to Section 2 symptoms

This item relates to the interference with normal, everyday activities and roles due to the presence of various symptoms in Section 2. Rate the actual degree of interference due to Section 2 symptoms using the scale in the manual.

ATTRIBUTIONS OF CAUSE

2.077   Organic cause of dissociative symptoms

Symptoms are characterized by a partial or complete disconnection between memories of the past, awareness of identity and immediate sensations, and control of bodily movements, but arising as a later consequence of an organic disorder.

General rules for rating attributions of cause are to be found in Section 13 of the Manual. Many items can be individually rated using the optional etiology scale. There should be an objective evidence for organic causation, and a temporal relationship between the underlying factor and the dissociative condition. The recovery of dissociative disorder should take place following improvement of the underlying presumed cause. The rating should be made on the basis of any dissociative symptoms rated present. The rating options allow the choice of uncertain, probable and definite judgements. Always `rate down'. The rating should be made at **2.078** and **13.034**. The nature of the cause can be recorded by means of the appropriate ICD-10 code in Section 13 at **13.049, 13.051, 13.053.**

2.078   Identify organic cause for Section 2 symptoms

2.080 - 2.135   Optional checklist of somatoform symptoms

See instructions above on page 24 of Glossary.

2.136   Relation of somatoform symptoms to panic attacks

Preoccupation with somatoform symptoms may occasionally occur in a similar time pattern to panic attacks (**4.020**) and for the purposes of classification it is necessary to rate whether these two forms of symptom presentation occur together.

3 Worrying, tension and other non-specific items

GENERAL POINTS ABOUT SECTION 3

Section 3 contains items that are often classified as 'neurotic'. 'Non-specific' is a better term, since most of them can occur alone, or in association with each other, and in the absence of more specific symptoms such as anxiety or depression. The latter disorders, on the other hand, are frequently accompanied by a range of non-specific dysfunctions. The non-specific items, and many neurotic items, tend to be characterized by three features that are frequently mentioned in the following definitions. They are painful experiences; they cannot be fully prevented or controlled by conscious effort; and in severity and persistence they are out of proportion to any circumstances that appear to precipitate them.

Many items can be understood as 'traits', i.e. they have been 'present' since adolescence or before. Symptoms (rated 1 to 3 according to severity) should only be rated if there has been an 'onset'; a definite departure from an earlier symptom-free state. See Rating Scale I for further details. However, if the date of definite onset can be established, it may be possible to record this at **3.014**, if most of the items in Section 3 follow that time course. If only one or two items have a protracted duration the date of the PERIOD should not be altered.

3.001 Worry

Perhaps the most ubiquitous psychiatric symptom, but with no diagnostic significance in itself. It demonstrates (regardless of content) three central principles that are characteristic of many non-specific and neurotic symptoms:

1 A round of painful, unpleasant or uncomfortable thought;
2 which cannot be consciously controlled by trying to turn the attention to subjects that would usually be absorbing;
3 and is often out of proportion to the topic worried about, so that the person affected appears consumed with worry about a triviality. Worry can be rated when the subject is painfully and uncontrollably concerned about a serious matter, like the death of a near relative, or the consequences of redundancy, but the interviewer should then be very sure that the worry is out of proportion; for example, it lasts longer than expected, or seriously impairs effective mental functioning. People may worry about their own mental state, or about their lack of energy or social inadequacy, or their psychotic experiences. The content of the worry is not relevant to recognition of its form.

The numerical rating requires the examiner's judgement as to how severe and how prolonged the worrying has been during the period under review.

Differentiation from other symptoms:

This symptom accompanies, and can be a precursor to, many others, such as hypochondriasis, depression, obsessions, and phobias, but it lacks their specific features. It occurs most commonly in the general population with other symptoms in Section 3 of PSE10; for example, muscular and nervous tension, exhaustion, and self-consciousness.

3.002 Subjective feeling of nervous tension

A feeling of inner restlessness or unease expressed in terms such as 'nerves', 'being on edge', 'being keyed up'. (Being 'up-tight' or 'wound-up' implies a degree of muscular tension as well and the two symptoms commonly co-exist.)

Nervous tension is a state of arousal that has three basic characteristics of many non-specific and neurotic symptoms - it is unpleasant, not under voluntary control and not fully explicable in situational terms. There is likely to be an exaggerated startle response. Autonomic symptoms such as are dealt with in Section 4 may or may not be frankly present; they are not a requirement for the symptom. Nervous tension is not linked to any particular mental content though it often does accompany symptoms such as worry and anxiety, and may appear as a precursor to them.

Differentiation from other symptoms:

'Muscular tension' (item **3.003**) is frequently present but it is not the same symptom and should be rated independently. Nervous tension should be differentiated from 'Anxiety' (item **4.023**) and 'Anxious foreboding' (item **4.024**), for which clear-cut autonomic symptoms must be present.

Normal situational nervousness, such as being keyed up before taking an examination, should be rated 0, not 1.

3.003 General muscular tension

An unpleasant tension in one or more groups of muscles, with inability to relax voluntarily. The muscular tension is not related to any specific intended muscular effort.

Almost any group of muscles can specifically be affected (see item **3.005**), but in the present item only general tension is rated. Rate on the basis of frequency and intensity during the past month.

Differentiation from other symptoms:

Muscular is differentiated from nervous tension, in that the latter is purely subjective. The two often go together, but they are different symptoms and should be rated separately.

Rate 9 if the tension is due to a physical cause, particularly the prescription of neuroleptic drugs.

3.004 Calmness in the face of problems

This item, like **2.001** and **6.004** and others, is included in order to allow people with few symptoms (e.g. in population samples) to express a positive rather than a purely negative evaluation of their mental functions. This can also be true of those with symptoms that do not exclude positive functioning in some areas. The items are also helpful in confirming cut-off points.

Note the unusual rating scale, which avoids the possibility of misleading default ratings of 0.

3.005 Localized tension pains

This symptom is 'muscular tension' (item **3.003**) localized to particular muscle groups. One of the commonest complaints is of headache like a 'band round the temples' or 'a weight pressing down on the head', due to tension in the muscles of the scalp. Those afflicted are often clear about the relationship of the headache to muscular (and nervous) tension. Write down the localization of the tension pains whenever this item is rated as present. Other common localizations are the back, the neck and the shoulders. Chest pain may also be due to muscular tension. Tension pains occurring only once or twice a month should be rated 1.

Differentiation from other symptoms:

Be careful to exclude migraine and other known causes of headache. If there is any doubt about a specific organic cause for the pain, rate 9 (if the pains are thought to have a specific cause), or 8 (if not known).

3.006 Subjectively described restlessness

Muscular tension (item **3.003**) expressed in motor activity. In moderate degree it is shown by fidgeting of various parts of the body and an inability to stay still. In severe degree it is expressed by pacing up and down, wandering about, inability to sit down for very long. Three common criteria for non-specific symptoms must be met - the restlessness is experienced as unpleasant, it is not under voluntary control, and it is inappropriate to the situation respondents find themselves in.

The rating of severity is based on the respondent's own account of frequency and intensity during the past month. If independently observed to be present during the past month or at interview, rate at item **22.016**.

Differentiation from other symptoms:

Restlessness (**22.016**), Agitation (**22.017**) and Overactivity (**22.018**) can be behavioral manifestations of subjective restlessness but they may also be associated with a feeling of energy and need not be subjectively unpleasant. They should be rated on the basis of observed behavior alone. Item **3.006** should only be rated from the respondent's subjective description.

The symptom must be distinguished from akathisia due to neuroleptic medication, which is also often subjectively unpleasant. If the respondent clearly and convincingly relates this restlessness to such medication, consider rating 9. Check by asking respondent to stand still for a while, something that is much more difficult in akathisia than in psychogenic restlessness. See also the guide to motor examination on page 187 of the Glossary.

3.007   Fatiguability and exhaustion

A symptom often accompanying, and in part due to, symptoms such as 'muscular tension' (**3.003**), 'restlessness' (**3.006**), and 'worrying' (**3.001**). It should be rated independently. Three common criteria for a non-specific symptom should be met: subjects experience the fatigue as unpleasant, they are unable voluntarily to overcome it and it is inappropriate to the situation they find themselves in. Thus tiredness and sleepiness at the end of a hard day's work, or due to the after-effect of influenza, would not count. The tiredness is essentially a sense of mental and physical fatigue; worn out, lethargic, heavy - not merely sleepy. It can, however, accompany chronic loss of sleep. The most intense form of the symptom is exhaustion.

Differentiation from other symptoms:

Although it is possible to fall asleep as the result of being immobilized by physical fatigue, the symptom should be distinguished from sleepiness, and still more from hypersomnia (see item **8.016**).

Excessive fatigue following exercise is rated at items **2.040, 2.041, and 2.042**. If the tiredness is due to a physical cause, including medication or a viral infection, rate 9.

3.008   Sensitivity to noise

The squeaking or grating noise that chalk sometimes makes on a blackboard has an unpleasant quality to which some people are particularly sensitive. A similar quality may accompany any undifferentiated noise, such as car or plane engines, or loud music. Even noises that many people would find tolerable may have this quality for some. The respondent may say 'noises go right through me', 'it jars on me', 'I cannot stand it when a plane goes over'. The experience is unpleasant and distracting, and leads to avoidance of noisy environments. Anticipation of unpleasant noise may be as distracting as the noise itself.

Be careful to consider the actual noise level experienced. A rating of (1) is used when there is an unequivocally higher sensitivity than normal but this does not interfere with everyday activities. A rating of (3) is reserved for extreme sensitivity to noises that most people would not find intolerable so that there is substantial interference with activities.

Differentiation from other symptoms:

The symptom is sensitivity to noise, not simply dislike of loud noises. Do not take other symptoms, such as irritability, into account. They should be rated independently.

If difficult to differentiate in a case of tinnitus, or hyperacusis due to middle ear disease, rate 8 or 9, or rate the phenomenon and use etiology option.

3.009   Irritability

Overreadiness to respond to minor annoyances; 'being on a short fuse'; 'boiling up inside'. The respondent usually recognizes that the response is excessive, out of proportion to the circumstances and difficult to control. The experience is unpleasant. Rate an increase in irritability during the chosen episode compared with respondent's norm.

If this is mainly subjective, without much external evidence, apart perhaps for a few minor domestic quarrels, rate (1). If it is shown by a frequently raised voice, shouting or a readiness to pick quarrels but without violence, rate (2). If there is loss of control, with pushing or hitting, rate (3). If there is no exacerbation associated with an episode of psychiatric disturbance, but an expression of the usual personality, rate 9 (not applicable). However, if symptoms throughout the Section appear to date back to early life, and fulfill the criteria of a symptoms during the PERIOD, rate presence and severity and consider rating the date of onset at **3.014**. Rate according to R's own account. Any evidence in the case records or from an informant of behavioral irritability or aggression, can be rated at **22.018** and/or **23.004**.

Irritability is regarded as an important symptom in depression and mania. If necessary the symptom should be reviewed again when Sections 6 and 10 are being used.

Differentiation from other symptoms:

Consider pathological response to alcohol (**11.027**), and if present rate using etiology option if it completely accounts for the behavior.

The following items **3.010, 3.011,** and **3.013** represent overvalued ideas i.e., they are ideas in which the individual has invested lot of emotion and they are in the forefront of the subject's psyche. Even though he recognizes that they are not true he cannot help feeling like that and perhaps even acts on them.

3.010   Simple ideas of reference

In its moderate form (rated 2), this symptom is indicated by self-consciousness. Those afflicted cannot help feeling that people take notice of them - in buses, in a restaurant, or in other public places - and that aspects of themselves that they would prefer not to be noticed are somehow publicly observable. The accompanying guilt or shame is out of proportion compared to any possible cause, which may be no more than a tendency to blush easily. They realize that such feelings originate within themselves but the insight is of little value. The experience may accompany depression but is not solely the result of the mood change.

In its severe form, R may complain of a feeling of being laughed at or criticized, perhaps because of some peccadillo that others seem to know about. Again, there is insight into the true nature of the symptom, but it tends to vary and reassurance is rarely fully effective.

If a respondent does, in fact, have some distinguishing physical characteristic that might cause notice, rate (9) unless the subject's distress and lack of control of the self-reference is out of proportion.

Differentiation from other symptoms:

Do not include delusions of reference (items **19.004, 19.010, 19.011**), in which respondents believe that events refer to them personally and have no insight into the origin of the self-reference within themselves. Differentiate from guilty ideas of reference, in which the context of depressive mood and content of guilt are primary. Distinguish also from social phobias (items **4.033 - 4.036**), which may co-exist and should be rated independently, and dysmorphophobia (item **16.011**), in which self-reference is based on a feeling that the afflicted person's features have changed in some way.

3.011 Suspiciousness

This symptom usually accompanies a disorder such as depression, hypomania, delusional psychosis, schizophrenia or cognitive impairment. However it should only be rated present if there is a degree of insight concerning its internal origin; either an attribution to a mood change or failing memory, or simply a knowledge that it has no (or insufficient) external justification. Severity depends on the extent to which insight is partial and on the behavior that occurs when it lapses. Item **23.010** should be rated if suspiciousness is rated in behavior at examination or reported in case records or by an informant during the past month.

Differentiation from other symptoms:

Suspicion may be regarded as a symptom in mania. If necessary it should be reviewed again when Section 10 is being used.

Differentiation from delusions of persecution should be made according to the criteria at the beginning of Section 19.

3.012 Depersonalization

The symptom is based on a detachment from, or loss of, the emotional coloring that accompanies the consciousness or perception of self. R retains a degree of insight, knows the condition is abnormal, and describes it in 'as if' terms. The experience is one of feeling unreal; as if acting a part rather than being spontaneous and natural; like being a sham or the shadow of a real person.

A more severe form of the symptom occurs when the respondent actually feels as if dead or living in some entirely different 'parallel world' that cannot interact with this one.

Differentiation from other symptoms:

The basic experience of depersonalization (emotional detachment from the perception of self) may occur as part of an anxiety state or panic state, characteristically terminating the anxiety. This should be rated separately or additionally at item **4.026**. It is also specified as an anxiety symptom in some diagnostic rules, and is therefore included at **4.014**.

Derealization is a related symptom in which events or objects or people in R's environment are experienced as unreal (items **16.006**, **16.007**). There are also delusional forms (**16.013**). Opportunity to rate these phenomena in more detail is provided in Section 16, where two further items are included to rate depersonalization itself (**16.008** and **16.009**). Section 16 should always be rated if there is any indication of perceptual abnormalities. The Glossary for Section 16 items should be consulted, because other perceptual abnormalities may mimic depersonalization.

The term 'depersonalization' is sometimes used to describe a delusion of influence or control. These symptoms are rated in Section 18 of SCAN and are not included in depersonalization.

3.013 Non-delusional jealousy

R is preoccupied with thoughts that a sexual partner is, or might be, being unfaithful, in spite of lack of evidence and assurances of fidelity. The degree of conviction varies, but it usually takes the form of doubt, with only fluctuating certainty. The agony of doubt can lead to determined attempts to resolve the uncertainty by seeking evidence, looking for stray hairs on clothing; inspecting diaries; secretly following the partner; trying to interpret whether stains found on underclothing are signs of illicit sexual activity.

Severity is rated according to the extent and nature of activities designed to end uncertainty.

Differentiation from other symptoms:

Since people who do have grounds for jealousy can behave in a similar way and the importance placed on infidelity varies between cultures and between sexes, caution should be used when making a rating. The most clear-cut signs of morbid jealousy are seen in the delusional forms. If there is any possibility of this, rating should be deferred until items **19.016** and **19.017**. The Glossary definition of item **19.016**, delusional jealousy, is relevant.

3.014 Dates of PERIOD of Section 3 symptoms

It should only be necessary to make a record here if the dates of symptoms in Section 3 are clearly different from those already recorded for PS (left hand rating boxes) or RE / LB (left hand boxes) in Section 1. For example, a respondent who has recently developed a depressive episode may also have had positive items in this section that began many years previously, possibly during childhood or adolescence.

3.015 Interference due to items rated in Section 3

This item is self explanatory and is important for certain classification systems and for descriptive purposes. It also makes clear that interference is rated separately.

ATTRIBUTIONS OF PHYSICAL AND OTHER CAUSES

Items in Section 3 may be present but in the judgement of the interviewer may be the result of a separate physical cause or drug. If this occurs, use the optional etiology boxes for items and/or the more general ratings in Section 13. Do not rate a symptom as absent simply because of a suspicion that a physical or other external factor may have contributed to it. The etiology option is designed to allow separate ratings of phenomenology and etiology. Many items in this Section may also follow directly on an adverse life event or psychosocial trauma. Make the appropriate rating of presence and severity in this Section. If there is doubt as to whether the symptom presence criteria are met, rate 8.

4 Panics, anxiety, and phobias

GENERAL POINTS ABOUT SECTION 4

The Section has two major parts; the first dealing with panic attacks (whether or not in phobic situations) and more generalized anxiety, the second with phobias (or phobic avoidance). The first two items, above the cut-off point, are probes for the two main types of symptom. As usual, the cut-off point is crossed if there is any doubt as to whether either type of symptom is present.

The anxiety subsection begins with a list of anxiety symptoms, which can be presented as a card or read out by the interviewer. This is followed by items representing various kinds of anxiety symptoms based on autonomic imbalance. The severity of each can be rated independently of the others. There is one course item (**4.025**). Such items are placed throughout the PSE10 text, and must always be rated if the interview goes beyond the cut-off point, since they are used for classification purposes by computer algorithms.

If there have been no anxiety symptoms during the period under review because R has avoided the situations that provoke them, there is a skip to the subsection on phobias. This begins with three lists representing situational, social and specific (simple) phobias, followed by items to rate the most severe example of each, items to measure degree of phobic avoidance and interference. Course items follow (all important for diagnostic algorithms).

4.001   General rating of anxiety

4.002   General rating of phobias

Probe questions which, together with any other information available, help determine whether the cut-off point should be passed.

4.003 - 4.019   Anxiety symptoms

This list of anxiety symptoms, when not clearly due to physical factors or to appropriate environmental circumstances, is the basis (albeit, occasionally, through attempts to avoid them) for the definition of panic attacks, free-floating anxiety, anxious foreboding and in some classification systems, phobias. Use optional etiology boxes if due to identifiable physical factors. The criteria for rating physical cause are very strictly laid down (Section 13) and it may be necessary to rate a general physical attribution of cause in Section 13.

4.020   Panic attacks

Panic attacks are discrete episodes of marked autonomic anxiety, with a sudden onset, building rapidly (within minutes) to a crescendo and a maximum point. They may occur against a general background of autonomic anxiety or emerge with no symptomatic precursors. An attack may last up to an hour but dissipate gradually. Both free-floating and phobic forms of anxiety may be characterized by panic attacks (see item **4.055**) and multiple ratings are then required.

Severity is rated in terms of frequency.

Differential definitions:

Sudden onsets chiefly with palpitations should raise the possibility of a paroxysmal tachycardia. Rate 9 if there is clearly only a physical cause of 'panics' or if the attacks end suddenly. If there is some possibility that physical factors do not entirely explain the symptom, rate its presence conservatively but consider the rating of organic or physical attribution in Section 13 at item **13.019**.

An attack described by R as panic but lasting more than an hour may be part of a more general anxiety state.

Panic attacks occurring only as a direct result of psychotic experiences are rated 5.

4.021   Enduring apprehension of a further panic attack

This item represents a special form of item **3.001**, worry, but the concern and the preoccupation is focused specifically on fear of developing a further attack or attacks in a respondent who has already had such attacks previously. Use Scale I.

4.022   Action to prevent or to end panic attack

Panic attacks may lead to an escape response. People who cannot get their breath may rush outside for air. Those with agoraphobia may leave the bus they are travelling on, or rush out of a supermarket. Those who are anxious when left on their own, or who have a phobia of spiders and find a large one in the kitchen, may phone their spouse or a friend, or go into a neighbor's house. Taking anxiolytic medication to try to abort an attack and not just prevent it would also be rated here.

4.023   Free-floating autonomic anxiety

The essential requirement for rating this item is a clear-cut autonomic state of the type listed in **4.003 - 4.019**, accompanied by an affect of fear or apprehension. The respondent may describe this in terms of nervous tension (item **3.002**), which can be regarded as the cognitive component of autonomic anxiety. But since it can occur without anxiety or autonomic symptoms, it should be rated independently.

Isolated autonomic symptoms, such as occasional palpitations in the absence of the affect of anxiety, are not included in this symptom. However, those afflicted are sometimes unable to describe their affect clearly, even when there is a range of anxiety or autonomic symptoms. Clinical judgement should be used.

The autonomic anxiety should be free-floating, that is, not exclusively tied to some external situation. A common occasion is when affected people are trying to go off to sleep and, with their ear pressed into the pillow, hear their heart beating. A minor change in rhythm may make them think their heart will stop. A subjective feeling of being unable to take a breath properly is another common occurrence. Sometimes the anxiety is triggered by worrying thoughts, returning whenever a particular topic intrudes into consciousness. Anxiety with autonomic symptoms tends to be prolonged (not meeting the criteria for panic, though the two symptoms can occur alternately) rather than fluctuating but brief episodes should be included. Severity is rated according to intensity and frequency during the relevant period.

Differentiation from other symptoms:

If the criteria for panic attacks (**4.020**) are also met, a separate rating should be made.

If anxiety reactions are confined to certain situations they should be rated under 'situational anxiety', 'social phobia' or 'specific phobia' (items **4.046, 4.049, 4.052**). 'Anxious foreboding', as defined in symptom **4.024** below, is a separate symptom, rated independently.

Do not include anxiety appropriate to the situation, e.g. going into battle, narrowly avoiding a traffic accident, realistic fear of punishment, anxiety before or during an examination.

Anxiety due to psychotic symptoms, e.g. that the subject is being hunted and may be killed, should be rated 5.

4.024   Anxious foreboding with autonomic symptoms

The subject fears that something dreadful is going to happen. The foreboding is accompanied by autonomic symptoms. It may occur in particularly concentrated form first thing in the morning, when those afflicted feel unable to face the day ahead. The sense of foreboding is primary. Those afflicted in this way cannot readily explain what they are afraid of, and any specific worries appear, if at all, as a secondary elaboration.

Severity is rated according to intensity and frequency during the period.

Differentiation from other symptoms:

Do not include simple free-floating anxiety (item **4.023**) unaccompanied by foreboding, or appropriate anxiety concerning real worries.

Distinguish from somatic depression, which is worst early in the day and may involve rumination over ruination or other future disaster. Then the affect and symptomatic context is predominantly one of depression; anxiety is secondary. However, each SCAN item should be rated on its merits, irrespective of background diagnostic judgements (unless otherwise specified in the text). If depression and anxiety are present together, rate both, and also item **6.022**.

4.025 Duration of free-floating anxiety

This item is included because some nosologies require symptoms to have been present for a specified length of time in order to qualify for inclusion in a category. Entering the number of months provides enough information to meet several such rules. If the item is left blank, the computer accepts the default option (00) and no classification of general anxiety can be made. Raters, therefore, should always be sure to fill in all relevant course items.

4.026 Depersonalization/derealization with anxiety

See item **3.012** for a definition of depersonalization. This may be associated with anxiety with autonomic symptoms. Occasionally a panic attack may terminate in a state of depersonalization. Only the conjunction of the two kinds of experience (which may alternate) is rated at item **4.026**.

Differentiation from other symptoms:

This item is different from, but can co-exist with, items **3.012** and **16.006 - 16.009**.

PHOBIAS

GENERAL POINTS ABOUT PHOBIAS

Phobias are irrational fears of particular situations or objects, exposure to which, or thoughts of which, produce autonomic symptoms that are not under conscious control and a tendency to avoid the stimulus. Some classification systems (i.e. DSM) do not require autonomic symptoms to have been present but do require other symptoms of worry, tension and apprehension, as in Section 3 symptoms. There is marked distress due to avoidance or anxiety symptoms. Symptoms are restricted to the feared situation or to anticipation of the feared situation.

4.027 - 4.032   Situational phobias (Agoraphobia)
4.046 - 4.048

The full form of the symptom consists of autonomic anxiety (defined as in item **4.023**, with symptoms from the list of items **4.003 - 4.019**), which is confined to certain situations or causes avoidance of these situations. A central element is fear of being alone, particularly among strangers, (often called agoraphobia). Examples are autonomic anxiety due to being alone in a confined or open space (buses, lifts, trains, cars, fields, squares, etc.), or in crowds, or collapsing when no help is near. These fears are exacerbated by a sense of being trapped and alleviated by a sense of being supported. If the symptom is present with nervous tension (item **3.002**) without a history of autonomic accompaniments, or non-autonomic anxiety, rate 1 (partial); with autonomic accompaniments the full symptom is rated 2, as defined above. The appropriate symptom must have been rated also in Section 3.

Differentiation from other symptoms:

Two types of situations are not included here but are rated separately. The first is autonomic anxiety occurring when R is obliged to interact with others (items **4.033** - **4.036** and **4.050**). The fear of crowds in agoraphobia is associated with a feeling of aloneness in an anonymous mass of people rather than the more personal fear in social phobias.

The second is autonomic anxiety due to very specific causes, such as fear of feathers, birds, spiders, insects, cats, etc. (item **4.045**). These two kinds of symptoms may co-exist with 'situational anxiety' (**4.027** - **4.032**) and then more than one rating will be necessary. Similarly, subjects may suffer from both 'free-floating autonomic anxiety' (item **4.023**) and 'situational anxiety', and both symptoms will then be rated as present.

4.033 - 4.036   Social phobias
4.049 - 4.051

The symptom consists of autonomic anxiety (defined as in item **4.023**, with symptoms from the list of items **4.003** - **4.019**), which is confined to certain situations or causes their avoidance. The central feature is anxiety under the scrutiny of others. In the extreme form, R may be unable to eat, drink, or write in public, or join any social group. In milder cases, R may feel uneasy speaking to a group of friends, for example at a social gathering, worry about blushing or trembling in public, or feel apprehensive about approaching strangers to ask for directions. Fear of speaking on the phone may be a relatively isolated symptom or a part of a more severe disturbance. If the symptom is present with nervous tension (item **3.002**) without a history of autonomic accompaniments, or non-autonomic anxiety, rate 1 (partial); with autonomic accompaniments the full form of the symptom is rated 2, as defined above.

Differentiation from other symptoms:

Those who merely feel anxious due to lack of practice in speaking formally in front of an audience should not be rated here.

Other 'situational anxiety' or 'specific phobias' (items **4.027** - **4.032**, **4.037** - **4.045**) may co-exist, but it is important to differentiate this particular symptom since it often occurs alone.

Rate fear of eating in public only when this is due to fear of scrutiny by others, not when it is due purely to the fear of eating as it sometimes is in anorexia nervosa.

4.037 - 4.045   Specific (simple, isolated) phobias
4.052 - 4.054

The symptom consists of autonomic anxiety (defined as in item **4.023**, with symptoms from the list of items **4.003** - **4.019**), which is confined to certain specific situations or objects, or cause their avoidance. These include mice, insects, snakes, cats, feathers, birds, etc., as detailed in items **4.037** - **4.045**. The anxiety may generalize - e.g. the subject may be unable to leave the house for fear of meeting a cat. This should still be rated under this item. If the symptom is present with nervous tension (item **3.002**) without a history of autonomic accompaniments, or non-autonomic anxiety, rate 1 (partial); with autonomic accompaniments the full form of the symptom is rated 2, as defined above.

Differentiation from other symptoms:

'Free-floating autonomic anxiety' (item **4.023**) may also be present, in which case it is rated in addition.

The fear of contracting disease, **4.043**, should be distinguished (a) from the delusional conviction of having an illness (items **2.039**, **19.031**, **19.032**); (b) from dysmorphophobia (item **16.011**) and delusions about appearance (item **16.012**); (c) from delusional explanations of somatic hallucinations (e.g. items **17.028**, **17.029**); (d) from obsessional actions associated with cleanliness and fears of contamination (item **5.004**). It can be difficult to distinguish between a phobia, an obsession and a delusion if R's description is not clear. Refer to the definitions of items cited and always use the rating of 8 if clinical judgement remains uncertain after adequate examination.

4.047 **Avoidance of most severe situational/ social/ specific anxiety provoking situations**
4.050
4.053

Probe for efforts or actions to avoid the most severe situational/ social/ specific phobias. The anxiety induced by the three types of situation varies from mild to intense. The more severe it is, the more respondents are likely to try to avoid the provoking stimuli. This item allows a rating of degree of overall behavioral avoidance and the distress and pain that this causes. Take into account the specific cultural setting. Rate even if nervous tension (item **3.002**) without a history of autonomic accompaniments, or anxiety without autonomic accompaniments are described. Use Scale I.

4.048 **Interference due to most severe situational/ social/ specific phobias**
4.051
4.054

These items refer to the interference with normal everyday activities, work and duties.

4.055 **Relation of panics to phobias**

4.056 **Age at first onset of panics or phobias**

4.057 **Phobias began after an episode of schizophrenia**

4.058 **Phobias began after episode of major affective disorder**

These four course items should always be completed if any part of Section 4 is used. Use all the information available, from the respondent, other informants, and case records, to make clinical judgements. If necessary, enter approximate age (say, within 5 years or so), since this is more useful than leaving the box blank.

4.059   Dates of PERIOD/S of Section 4 symptoms

Record only if different from records in Section 1.

4.060   Interference with activities due to panic or autonomic anxiety symptoms

Use interference scale as in manual.

4.061   Organic cause of anxiety symptoms

Rating of phenomenology should in general be made without consideration of etiology. The etiology option allows individual items to be separately linked to an etiological attribution. This item allows a more general rating of **Section 4**.

Section 13 (item **13.019**) also allows a simple rating of whether an 'organic' cause is present, whether or not it can be specified in terms of an ICD-10 class.

4.062   Identify organic cause for Section 4 symptoms

Several organic conditions (for example, hyper- and hypothyroidism, pheochromocytoma and hypoglycemia, are known to be accompanied by symptoms of anxiety. The letter identifying the ICD-10 chapter, and up to three digits, should be entered here and/or in Section 13. A list is provided in the Appendix.

Psychoactive substances rated in Sections 11 and 12, such as alcohol, cocaine, amphetamines and sedatives, can cause anxiety symptoms as toxic or as withdrawal effects.

5 Obsessional symptoms

GENERAL POINTS ABOUT SECTION 5

The term 'obsession' is used, for convenience, to cover 'compulsions' as well.

The central feature of the subjective component of these symptoms is that they are experienced as occurring against conscious resistance i.e., they are intrusive and ego dystonic. In the case of compulsions, this is accompanied by expression in behavior. After a very long time the experience of conscious resistance may begin to lose its force if R habitually yields to the impulse - but the nature of the symptoms is by then quite obvious. They are recognized as being part of the respondent's own thoughts, and have an unpleasant repetitive quality. If some elements of the symptom are missing - for instance, habitual tidiness without a sense of compulsion - and there has been no 'onset', consider the possibility that this is a life long trait and part of the respondent's personality. If uncertain, rate 8. Do not rate items present in Section 5 if a trait explanation suffices.

Differentiation from other symptoms:

The criteria given above apply to all Section 5 phenomena. Fear of contracting disease (item **4.043**) should be distinguished from an obsessional preoccupation with contamination from germs and the accompanying compulsions. Hypochondriacal delusions (items **2.039, 19.027, 19.028**) carry no subjective experience of resistance. Tourette's Syndrome should be rated 9, but only if the examiner is certain that obsessional phenomena cannot be differentiated (both forms of disorder existing together should be considered). The symptom must also be differentiated from worry which is not recognized by the subject as intrusive even though it may in fact be unpleasant.

Occasionally obsessions have or develop features characteristic of delusions - one woman became delusionally convinced that there really was a baby stuck down the toilet, whereas before she had merely experienced obsessional doubt. In such cases the delusion should be rated in preference, since the phenomenology has changed. In other cases, subjects may claim to have heard voices, as with a woman who could not travel past a graveyard because she thought that people had been buried alive and she felt impelled to make sure that they had not - the voice confirmed her fears and in the process she moved from obsessional doubt to delusional conviction.

The differentiation from obsessional traits can be difficult. It is particularly important to be sure that there has been a clear onset following a period with no symptoms, or a marked exacerbation from a previous steady state.

The rating scale omits a code of 1, because of the necessity to ensure that the symptom really is present and not part of the normal range of variation in traits such as orderliness, indecisiveness or carefulness.

5.001   Evidence for obsessional and compulsive symptoms

Because of the extensive probing for symptoms in this Section, there is only one item above the cut-off point. An entry of 0 indicates that the interviewer is satisfied that no obsessional or compulsive symptoms are present.

5.002   Obsessional checking and repeating

The checking or repetitive action is experienced as being carried out against conscious resistance. Such respondents are impelled to check light switches or gas taps many times (not just two or three times), to touch or count things, or to repeat the same action over and over again. Sometimes the repetition has a ritual quality designed to control the feared situation in a superstitious way. Respondents know that the compulsion comes from within themselves.

5.003   Obsessional actions associated with excessive orderliness

Those afflicted are not merely tidy; their tidiness is associated with a precise arrangement or ordering of objects - for example, currency notes must be the right way round in the wallet; jackets must face the same way in the wardrobe; actions have to follow a rigid sequence, for instance, in preparing for sleep. If such compulsions are not obeyed, there is a strong sense of unease, anxiety, irritability or distress. At the same time, it is recognized that these are internal compulsions. Include eating and cooking rituals.

5.004   Obsessional thoughts of harm or accidents

These ideas enter the mind against conscious resistance. Respondents are impelled to think of certain (usually unpleasant and distressing) ideas or images, such as knives or obscenities. They may, for example, have the urge to plunge knives into people who are with them, or to harm them in other ways. They recognize this impulse as emerging from within themselves, but are distressed because the thoughts are at variance with how they normally view themselves. One mother had the repetitive thought about her much loved new baby 'I wish she were dead.' Such thoughts may be associated with controlling compulsions or rituals, e.g. hiding knives away, thinking three good thoughts in a row, etc. It may be appropriate to rate item **5.001** in addition.

Because the thoughts are usually unacceptable to respondents, they may sometimes describe them as alien. By this they mean alien to their personal views and attitudes. Further questioning will elicit the acknowledgement that, however distasteful, they do not lack the sense of possession over their thoughts. The item can thus be distinguished from thought insertion (item **18.006**).

5.005   Obsessional actions associated with cleanliness

The preoccupation with contamination and the associated rituals to prevent it occurring, such as excessive handwashing, are experienced against conscious resistance. Respondents with the symptoms recognize that they are senseless and do their best, at least in the early stages, to resist them, but cannot. They are compelled to wash, or to avoid touching things in fear of contamination, or to carry out other complex rituals to do with cleanliness, over and over again.

5.006 Obsessional rumination and feelings of incompletion

Those affected experience repetitive and intrusive thoughts against conscious resistance. These are often to do with an attempt at finding the answer to some problem or getting some abstruse subject clear in their minds. They may have to convince themselves that they have remembered every detail of a particular event. They may have to ruminate endlessly and inconclusively about some philosophical theory. Sometimes they may have to rehearse in their mind the details of a task they cannot convince themselves they have completed. If a good description of such difficulties is spontaneously provided by R, rate (2). At its most severe, the processes of thought and speech are vague, repetitive, tortuous and pointless, but must be continued nevertheless. Rate (3) on the basis of a speech disorder that clearly reveals the underlying phenomenon.

Differentiation from other symptoms:

This disorder, when chronic and without subjective resistance or apparent distress, should be distinguished from 'drivelling' or 'rambling' speech (item **24.007**), by the fact that it develops from characteristic obsessional beginnings.

5.007 Fading of conscious resistance to obsessional symptoms

The typical obsessional experience involves ideas that intrude against conscious, and often desperate, attempts to exclude them. This is one of the key elements in recognizing the nature of the symptom. However, after many years of struggle, the resistance may begin to fade and even disappear entirely, although respondents seldom forget the strength of their initial reaction.

This item is included to record such fading and to allow a classification even if it has occurred.

5.008 Relation of anxiety to obsessional symptoms

5.009 Relation of depressive to obsessional symptoms

5.010 Relation of obsessions to compulsions

5.011 Insight into obsessions and or compulsions

Those affected by repetitive and unpleasant thoughts, ideas and images and compulsions usually acknowledge that these originate in their mind and are not imposed by outside persons or influences. Their efforts to resist them are unsuccessful to a varying extent. Those affected also acknowledge that the obsessions and compulsions are excessive and unreasonable. Probe the extent to which respondent recognizes that obsessions and/or compulsions are unreasonable and excessive and rate using the Scale.

5.012 Content of obsessional symptoms limited to another disorder

The obsessional thoughts, ideas or images may be the result of other mental disorders such as mood disorders, hypochondriasis or schizophrenia and related disorders. Rate here the extent to which content of obsessional symptoms are limited to another disorder.

5.013 Age at first onset of obsessional symptoms

These three course items should always be completed if any part of Section 5 is used. Use all the information available, from the respondent, other informants, and case records, to make clinical judgements.

5.014 Dates of PERIOD/S of obsessional symptoms

Use only if different from dates in Section 1, i.e. if obsessional symptoms have begun in childhood and other symptoms more recently.

5.015 Interference with activities due to Section 5 symptoms

The obsessions and/or compulsions usually cause varying degrees of distress and interference with the respondents social or individual functioning and everyday activities. Rate the degree to which Section 5 symptoms cause interference with daily activities using the Scale provided.

5.016 ATTRIBUTIONAL RATINGS (See Also Section 13)
5.017

Rating of phenomenology should in general be made without consideration of etiology. The etiology option allows individual items to be separately rated for an etiological attribution. At the syndromal or section level a rating of whether an 'organic' cause is present, whether or not it can be specified in terms of an ICD-10 class can be made here and/or at item **13.020** in Section 13. Rules for making such attributions of cause can be found in the manual and glossary, Section 13.

Tourette's syndrome may be associated with obsessional symptoms, in which case it can be entered there. The letter identifying any ICD-10 chapter, and up to three digits (see Appendix), should be entered also in Section 13.

6   Depressed mood and ideation

GENERAL POINTS ABOUT SECTION 6

In general symptoms of affective disorder have a clear-cut onset. However, if duration is very longstanding, there are opportunities to record the relevant dates in this Section.

6.001   Depressed mood

Depressed mood may be expressed in a number of ways - sadness, misery, low spirits, inability to enjoy anything, gloom, dejection, feeling blue. There are innumerable local variants, with which examiners should be familiar. Depression may sometimes be expressed as apathy but this should be excluded from the present rating unless there is good evidence, for example if it is a development from frank depression. Depressive apathy may be included in the rating of 'masked depression' (item **6.003**) or 'depression on examination' (item **23.002**). Tearfulness, which should be rated separately (item **6.004**), is a clue to severity, although it is neither sufficient nor necessary (the deepest depression may be a frozen misery which is beyond tears). Another criterion of severity is lack of variability (or in other words loss of reactivity); moderate forms of depression tend to come and go more than severe forms. Occasional sadness is part of normal human experience. It becomes pathological when it is persistent, pervasive, unresponsive, painful and out of proportion. It should then be rated as present even if there has been an apparently sufficient cause.

Criteria for rating (1)

Brief episodes of clinically depressed mood may occur on their own or appear within episodes of elated affect. A criterion for a rating of 1 is a period lasting at least 2 days. Mood changes of briefer duration should be included if repeated several times. If rated 1, always proceed beyond the cut-off point. This is an exception to the usual rule in Part One.

Criteria for rating (2)

The intensity is variable; the depression is sometimes not very severe or even absent. There may sometimes be deep depression but for brief periods of a few hours only. Occasional episodes of crying may occur, often because of some upsetting incident. Respondents cannot switch attention voluntarily to non-depressing topics, but it can be directed temporarily to pleasanter matters (for example, by working hard, by the conversation of others, by chance happenings of an interesting kind). If a major loss such as a bereavement has occurred the severity, duration or intensity should be unusual under the circumstances during the PERIOD. The examiner should consider how many people would feel this way under these circumstances and rate 2 if the mood is unusual, but rate 1 if within the generally expected range.

The depression remains in the background and tends to come flooding back. In most cases, depression of this degree should last 14 days or more to be rated (2), but mood changes of briefer duration should be included if repeated several times. Duration of depressed mood is rated separately in item **6.002**.

Criteria for rating (3)

Deep depression lasts for long periods of time without variation unless it is regularly diurnal. There are episodes of crying for no reason at all, unless there is apathy or approaching stupor. The mind is almost totally occupied by depressing topics; it is very difficult for the subject to give attention to anything else, e.g. cannot be distracted by working harder, watching something interesting on the television, or other people's conversation. Depression of this degree will almost certainly last 14 days or more to be rated (3). Depression of this severity can occur following a major loss or trauma but will be clearly excessive and out of keeping with the circumstances.

Differentiation from other symptoms:

Other forms of unpleasant affect (e.g. worrying, nervous tension, or anxious foreboding) should be rated separately (see definitions for items **3.001**, **3.002** and **4.024** respectively). Depression may well be present at the same time.

If present on and off for two years or more, consider rating also the checklist on dysthymia.

6.002 **Duration of depressed mood**

This item is self explanatory. It is essential for certain classification systems. Differentiate from **6.026** (dates of the whole range of depressive symptoms).

6.003 **Masked depression**

This item is included to provide for circumstances when respondents cannot be rated as overtly depressed (or not at an appropriate level of severity) but the interviewer considers that the depression is masked. The possibilities are:

(a) Another mood, such as irritability, in which case do not rate here but at item **3.009**;
(b) Apparent flatness of mood due to a loss of the capacity to feel sadness or other emotions that have been present, (see item **6.007**);
(c) Difficulty with introspection, because of cognitive problems or language difficulties;
(d) Educational problems;
(e) Local cultural tendency to manifest depression in forms other than mood, e.g. in somatic symptoms;
(f) Denial.
(g) Mistrust or suspiciousness.

Rate whether masked depression is possibly (1) or probably (2) present. In either case always proceed beyond the cut-off point.

6.004 Tearfulness and crying

Tears as an immediate response to an upsetting event are not pathological. Occasional but overt weeping over a period of days should be rated 2, even in the context of an understandable provocation, if the criteria for non-specific symptoms stated at the head of Section 3, above, are met. Long periods of weeping, without any control, are rated 3.

Note an inability to weep may suggest very severe depression but is not rated at this item.

If present on and off for two years or more, consider rating the checklist on dysthymia.

6.005 Capacity for enjoyment

Respondents with this symptom lose the ability to take pleasure in activities that normally provide it. They are also no longer capable of pleasurable anticipation. In order to rate 3 or 4, there must have been an identifiable change from an earlier, happier, state.

This item, like **2.001, 3.004** and others, is included in order to allow people with few symptoms (e.g. in population samples) to express a positive rather than a purely negative evaluation of their mental functions. This can also be true of those with symptoms that do not exclude positive functioning in some areas. The items are helpful in confirming cut-off points.

A rating of 1 is reserved for people who are positively enjoying their circumstances and activities during the period under consideration. Confine the present rating to the enjoyment of activities that would ordinarily be found pleasurable by the respondent.

Note the unusual rating scale, which avoids the possibility of misleading default ratings of 0.

If present on and off for two years or more, consider rating the checklist on dysthymia.

CUT-OFF POINT

Always continue below the cut-off point if there is any reason to suppose that any of the remaining Section 6 items are present. Remember that some of them could be present in the absence of depressed mood. If Section 6 symptoms are present, extra care should be taken to check for Section 7 and 8 symptoms.

6.006 Loss of hope for the future

The afflicted person's view of the future is bleak and without comfort, irrespective of the true circumstances. A judgement on clinical severity turns on the extent to which there is an attempt to cope, or islands of some hope (rating of 2), or whether personal and social affairs are neglected because of hopelessness about the future. Hopelessness is a common accompaniment and apparent cause of suicidal thoughts and behavior but these should be rated separately. Note that hopelessness is not necessarily accompanied by depression. Use the three criteria stated at the head of Section 3 above.

Differentiation from other symptoms:

Delusions with content centered on ruination, disease and death may or may not be accompanied by a feeling of hopelessness. Insofar as it is possible, the feeling should be rated separately from the content. Use a rating of 5 if the separation cannot be made.

If present on and off for two years or more, consider rating the checklist on dysthymia.

6.007   **Feeling of loss of feeling**

The respondent must describe a definite **loss** of the ability to feel emotion, compared with their normal state. The description in Eugen Bleuler's textbook is: 'The loss of feeling is felt, the numbness perceived, the lifelessness experienced'. Respondents can remember a time when they did have the capacity for feeling, which might have been months or years earlier. The symptom need not have begun during the period being rated. An example is an elderly depressed woman who can no longer feel the love she had (and says she still has) for her grandchildren. The inability to feel this love causes severe distress.

The symptom is usually associated with depressed mood, particularly if there is chronic depressive apathy. It can also be associated with irritability and with affects such as anxiety. Respondents may also say they are depressed, meaning that an earlier mood of sadness has been replaced by numbness or that the two symptoms are present together.

Differentiation from other symptoms:

This is a subjective complaint and should not be confused with blunting of affect (item **23.008**). The symptom is not delusional, and it is not lack of insight. There is no equivalent trait since the symptom must have an onset.

6.008   **Unremitting depression**

The rating depends solely on the unchanging nature of the depressed mood. Rate 3 if depression is pervasively present, even if there is some variation in intensity with circumstances. See Scale in Manual for further instructions.

6.009   **Morning depression**

The respondent states unequivocally that depression is worst during the early part of the day and then improves. Characteristically, subjects wake early and then lie awake feeling that they cannot get up and face the day. There may be a marked sense of speeding up as the day progresses, with a return even to normal mood by evening. Rate this (1).

If depression is not particularly marked in mornings, or is marked both in the mornings and the evenings, rate (0).

6.010   Preoccupation with death or catastrophe

This item is rated on the content of depressive preoccupations that fall short of delusional quality. This may involve physical damage, domestic upset, financial disaster, or illness that may happen to respondents, or to members of their families or friends. They realize the thoughts originate within themselves, and can achieve some objectivity concerning the real situation. Nevertheless, the ideas have a powerful hold on the imagination. Where a belief in the fact or certainty of specific disasters is held with unshakable conviction, rate under item **6.019 / 19.026.**

If present on and off for two years or more, consider rating the checklist on dysthymia.

6.011   Suicide or self-harm

A rare and fleeting thought about suicide is not rated here. Persistent intrusiveness or a more deliberate consideration or planning of possible techniques is rated (1). If a suicidal act is actually made, including a moderate degree of self injury, but there is doubt as to whether it was really intended to result in the Respondent's death, rate (2). Serious self-harm under similar circumstances is rated (3.) A definite attempt, clearly intended to result in death is rated (4), irrespective of the degree of self harm that followed. Seriousness of intent can be judged from R's knowledge of how lethal the method was, attempts to avoid discovery and behavior indicating a belief that the attempt would be successful e.g. a suicide note.

Note that ratings of this item do not require an assumption that depressed mood was the cause of the behavior.

6.012   Tedium vitae

The respondent states that life holds nothing of interest and that there appears no positive reason for continuing it. The feeling lacks the active, intrusive quality of suicidal ideation, but there may be a strong wish, passively expressed, not to wake in the morning, to welcome the idea of a fatal disease, and perhaps even seek an accident.

6.013   Pathological guilt

Overconcern with some action that most people would agree was blameworthy is usually rated (1). It can be given a higher rating, if it is painful, out of proportion and beyond control. For a rating of (2) pathological guilt can take two forms. In one form, respondents blame themselves too much for some peccadillo which most people would not take very seriously. They realize that the guilt is exaggerated or unduly prolonged, but cannot help feeling it all the same. The second form of moderate pathological guilt may concern actions or deficiencies that have some basis in fact. However, respondents experience a sense of guilt that is painful and excessive. Respondents are aware (perhaps with occasional lapses) that the feeling is out of proportion to circumstances. Rate this condition (2), irrespective of frequency during the relevant period.

In the more intense form of the symptom, respondents generalize the feeling of self-blame to almost anything that goes wrong in their environment. They realize that the guilt is exaggerated but cannot help feeling it all the same. Rate this condition (3) irrespective of frequency during the period. Do not include delusions of guilt in which subjects feel they have committed some terrible crime or are to blame for all the sins of the world, and have no insight into the origins of the symptom within their own minds (items **6.018** / **19.025**).

6.014 Guilty ideas of reference

The characteristics of 'simple ideas of reference' (item **3.010**) are present, but the feeling is based on guilt in the context of depressed mood. Respondents feel that they are blamed for some action or attribute. They realize that this feeling originates within themselves, but cannot help feeling it all the same, quite out of proportion to any possible cause. Rate this condition as (2), irrespective of frequency during the past month.

In the more intense form of the symptom, subjects actually feel that they are accused of some blameworthy action or attribute. Again they realize that this feeling originates within themselves but cannot help feeling it all the same. Rate this condition as (3), irrespective of frequency during the past month.

If the subject has actually committed some blameworthy act this may be rated in the usual way, provided only that other people cannot know of it. If they do know of it, rate 9.

Differentiation from other symptoms:

Do not include delusions of guilt (items **6.018** / **19.025**) in which respondents think they deserve punishment for some crime that they have committed. Do not include pathological guilt, not amounting to delusions, which is not projected as an idea of reference (item **6.013**). Other differentiations are from dysmorphophobia (item **16.011**) and its delusional form (item **16.012**), and social phobias (particularly items **4.035** and **4.036**).

6.015 Loss of self-confidence with other people

Afflicted people lose confidence in their social skills and anticipate discomfort and failure in matters which depend upon confidence in social relationships. Do not take into account confidence in mechanical or intellectual abilities. The loss may be caused by the presence of other mental symptoms, such as depression, which are rated separately.

Differentiation from other symptoms:

It is particularly important to rate the symptom only on the basis of a definite **loss** of normal functioning. Poor self-confidence can occur as a life-long trait and be accompanied by, and possibly cause, depression. Since this does not meet the criteria for a symptom it should be rated absent, or uncertain (8).

Other possibly confusing symptoms are ideas of reference (item **3.010**); social phobias (particularly items **4.035, 4.036**); guilty ideas of reference (item **6.014**); dysmorphophobia (item **16.011**). These are all possible accompaniments or causes and should be rated separately.

If present on and off for two years or more, consider rating the checklist on dysthymia.

6.016 Social Withdrawal

In the less intense form of the symptom, R does not seek company but does not refuse it when offered. In the more intense form, the subject actively withdraws and refuses company even when it is offered. Rate severity on a combination of severity and intensity.

Differentiation from other symptoms:

If social withdrawal appear to be a life-long 'trait' consider also the rating of Hypersensitivity to Interpersonal rejection (item **27.034**). Differentiate also from social phobia and avoidance of social phobia (items **4.033 - 4.036** and **4.050**) and from Suspiciousness (item **3.011**).

The commonest accompanying mental state is depression, which may be a cause or a consequence and should be rated independently.

6.017 Self-depreciation

Respondents with this symptom say that they feel inferior to others, even - in the most intensive form of the symptom - worthless. Ideas of self-depreciation are an exaggerated form of self-knowledge about part of the subject's own character, which gives a false picture because it is not counter-balanced by a recognition that most human beings have similar faults. Self-depreciation implies a raising of the standard applied to the subject without an equivalent raising of the standard applied to others, or taking into account balancing merits.

The commonest accompanying mental state is depression, which may be a cause or a consequence and should be rated independently.

Differentiation from other symptoms:

Distinguish from symptoms such as guilt (item **6.013**), ideas of reference (items **3.010**, **6.014**) social phobias (items **4.035, 4.036**), and depressive delusions of guilt (item **6.018 / 19.025**).

If present on and off for two years or more, consider rating the checklist on dysthymia.

6.018
6.019   **Psychotic phenomena associated with depression**
6.020
6.021

These items are repeated in Part II of SCAN at items **19.025, 19.026, 19.027** and **17.010, 17.011** respectively. They are defined there. If ratings are made in Section 6, the computer program allocates them to their equivalents in Part II. If both sets of items are rated, the Part II items are given preference. It should be noted that other relevant psychological and behavioral abnormalities are rated only in Part II, for example, stupor (item **22.006**). If there is any doubt as to whether to proceed to Part II, always do so. A few relevant items (e.g. depressed affect on examination, items **14.015 / 23.002**) will be found in the Screen, Section 14, but this is intended for Stage 1 population surveys, not for clinical examination.

6.022   **Depression or anxiety primary**

If the subject suffers from both anxiety and depression, and both have been rated as being present, try to decide which is primary. Respondents are quite often clear about the answer; however, the judgement must be made by the interviewer on the basis of all the available information.

Anxiety is primary when any depression appears to be mainly explicable in terms of the limitations placed on respondents by their anxiety symptoms, or seems part of the anxiety process. Thus being unable to leave home or travel or meet people, or being afraid that palpitations mean heart disease, may be very depressing. Respondents may be clear, however, that if the anxiety symptoms were not present the depression would vanish also. On the other hand, the anxiety might well remain even if the depression disappeared. These situations, or when long-standing anxiety provides a context for intermittent and probably derivative depression, are rated (1).

At the other extreme, the symptoms of anxiety may be reactive to the depressive condition - particularly if anxiety takes the form of fears of catastrophe, forebodings about illness or death, early morning dread at having to face the day, or a feeling that something awful is going to happen. In other cases the anxiety can be seen as part of a depressive process. Even when there are autonomic accompaniments, these anxiety symptoms may be seen quite clearly as secondary to depression - they would disappear if the depression did, but the depression would not necessarily be better if the anxiety disappeared. Anxiety due to fear of morbid or suicidal ideas is even more clearly secondary to depression. These conditions are rated (3).

In between these two fairly straightforward conditions, there are situations in which both anxiety and depression are present, but either they seem independent of each other or it is not possible to decide which one is primary. Rate both of these conditions (2).

There is a full definition of rating levels in the PSE10 text. The item is not used in algorithms but is useful for research into the relationship between anxiety and depressive disorders.

6.023   Relation of somatoform to depressive symptoms

These course items should always be completed if any part of Section 6 is used. Use all the information available, from the respondent, other informants, and case records, to make clinical judgements.

6.024   Relation of obsessional to depressive symptoms

These course items should always be completed if any part of Section 6 is used. Use all the information available, from the respondent, other informants, and case records, to make clinical judgements.

6.025   Age at first onset of depressive symptoms

6.026   Dates of PERIOD/S of depressive symptoms

Apply the same principles as set out in Section 3. Only record if absolutely necessary.

6.027   Interference with activities due to depression

This item relates to the ability to carry out normal activities and roles, which tends to be progressively impaired as depression deepens. Some people are affected at relatively moderate levels of depression, others soldier on until there is a precipitate collapse of function. Rate actual performance, as indicated in the scale.

6.028   Organic cause of Section 6 depressive symptoms

Rating of phenomenology should in general be made without consideration of etiology. The etiology option allows individual items to be separately rated for an etiological attribution.

6.029   Identify organic cause for Section 6 depressive symptoms

Rating of whether an 'organic' cause is present, whether or not it can be specified in terms of an ICD-10 class should be considered and rated here and/or in Section 13 or using the etiology option for individual items.

Endocrine disorder, dementia or other physical disorders associated with depressive symptoms may be recorded in Section 13. The letter identifying the ICD-10 chapter, and up to three digits, should be entered. A list is provided in the Appendix.

Psychoactive substances rated in Sections 11 and 12, such as alcohol and cocaine, can cause depressive symptoms as toxic or as withdrawal effects (**11.019** and **12.034**).

6.030   Episodes of major affective disorder

6.031   Personality before onset

6.032   Severity of affective episodes

6.033   Two or more depressive episodes with recovery

6.034   Response to adequate antidepressant therapy

6.035   One or more manic episode during the course

These course items should always be completed if any part of Section 6 is used. Use all the information available, from the respondent, other informants, and case records, to make clinical judgements.

6.036   Mixed episodes during the episode of illness

A mixed episode is characterized by either a mixture or a rapid alternation of hypomanic or manic with depressive symptoms. Rate 3 if the current episode is mixed.

6.038 - 6.043   Dates of 6 most recent episodes of depressive disorders before PE

This rating is required for the classification of ICD-10 and DSM diagnoses of recurrent, seasonal and rapid cycling subtypes of depression. If clear-cut episodes have occurred with remissions shorter than the usual period (defined in SCAN as 2 months) their dates should still be recorded as separate episodes. The algorithms will deal with these data subsequently, depending on the classification rules being applied. Definitions of onset and remission (quality of remissions **1.018**) are as in Section 1 of the Glossary and should be re-rated if necessary having completed Sections 6 and 10.

6.044 - 6.061   Persistent Depressive States, Dysthymia

This is an optional checklist but it can be rated using information collected during other parts of the interview and should therefore be completed if there is any possibility that the disorder may be present.

There is persistent despondency or gloom lasting at least 2 years, with basic coping and periods of normal mood, but with a general feeling of insufficiency. Poor sleep, low energy, tedium vitae, and brooding are common.

Most of the symptoms involved can be considered when rating other items in Part One of SCAN. They are identified by a line reading, 'If > 2 years consider dysthymia'. The ratings of dysthymic symptoms should only be made at Checklist items **6.044 - 6.061**.

Since it will often not be clear, before the interview begins, whether the symptoms have lasted for more than 2 years and whether the other course criteria apply, the appropriate strategy is to make general enquiries about the course at the beginning of Section 6 and then complete the relevant Sections 6, 7 and 8. (Some items in Section 3 are also of relevance.) If R is clearly in an episode of major depression it is not necessary to complete the dysthymia Checklist, except for research purposes. (The status of the disorder will be clarified by co-morbidity studies.)

If in doubt, complete both Section 6 and Checklist, as the computer program will appropriately classify cases which do in fact meet criteria for the various depressive conditions.

Note that most of the dysthymic symptoms also occur in cyclothymia (Checklist items **10.031 - 10.050**). It may be convenient to complete both Checklists at the same time.

6.072 - 6.074   Recurrent brief depressive disorder

So far as the interview is concerned, similar recommendations apply to this Checklist as to those for dysthymia and cyclothymia. The disorder meets criteria for depressive episode and it is sensible, therefore, to complete the relevant main sections of Part One.

It is necessary to bear the course criteria in mind when conducting the interview. There should be a phase at least once a month during the previous year, phases should usually last a few days only, and they should not occur only in association with the menstrual cycle.

7 Thinking, concentration, energy and interests

GENERAL POINTS ABOUT SECTION 7

Symptoms in Section 7 are grouped together for convenience but it will often be necessary to take them out of order, for example when rating a depressive episode or dysthymia. However, all can (and in population surveys do) occur without being part of any specific mental or physical disorder. Depression is not the only disorder associated, though it is probably the commonest. Psychotic or cognitive impairments are other prominent associations; Part II should always be rated if they are suspected.

Be particularly careful to eliminate any tendency to rate items present according to presuppositions as to the eventual diagnosis. This Section is concerned only with the extent of any loss of efficiency at carrying out the functions specified.

Items must also be rated according to the general rule that distinguishes between SYMPTOMS (with a definite onset following a period without the characteristic) and traits (which have 'always' been present). Thus 'loss' does not necessarily mean during the past month or some other restricted period of time that is being rated. It means a loss compared with a previous state, which has persisted into the period under review. For example, if an episode of depression began 2 years ago, and loss of interest dates from that time and is still present, include it in PS. The extent of loss during the episode is compared with the usual level of interests before the loss. Lifelong lack of interest may be thought of as a personality trait (which cannot be rated as a symptom). If in doubt, rate 8. However, the 'onset' of such 'complaints' can sometimes be dated back to a clearly recalled time in childhood and if the criteria for a symptom rating can be made, the date of onset can be recorded for the PERIOD at item **7.008**.

7.001 Positive cognitive functioning

This item, like items **2.001, 3.004** and **6.005**, provides a useful indication as to whether to use the cut-off, and also an opportunity to rate positive functioning independently of other items where impaired functioning is recorded. Someone who is depressed, for example, may nevertheless be able, through determined concentration, to exploit talents or skills efficiently. This may also allow attention to be turned away from painful subjective experiences. As everywhere in the SCAN schedules, interviewers are asked to rate each item according strictly to the definition, independently of any expectations derived from other ratings.

The item is rated following general probes concerning the functions covered. Note the unusual rating scale.

CUT-OFF POINT

If Section 6 symptoms are present, be particularly careful to consider all Section 7 items.

7.002   Loss of Concentration

Those affected complain that they cannot give full attention to matters that require it, or not for as long as is required. The experience is unpleasant, it is beyond the subject's power to correct except for very brief intervals, and it is out of proportion to the difficulty of the problems being considered. At its most intense, subjects cannot even read a few sentences in a newspaper, cannot watch television, and cannot take part in a conversation because their mind wanders off.

If subjects are definitely aware of a reduction in their normal ability to concentrate, but the effects are minimal, rate (1). If the symptom is causing moderate impairment in functioning, e.g. an ability to take in written material for adequate periods or without considerable subjective effort, rate (2). The severity criterion for rating (3) is that at which the subject is virtually unable to take things in at all.

Differentiation from other symptoms:

There may be several reasons for poor concentration, including worrying, inefficiency of thinking, distractibility, anxiety, delusions, etc. The rating should be made on the basis of whether the symptom is present, not on what its cause is.

If a respondent has thought insertion, commentary, withdrawal or broadcast (items **18.005 - 18.011**), or other psychotic experiences or explanations, or thought or speech disorder, that make the rating difficult, rate (5).

If present on and off for two years or more, consider rating the checklist on dysthymia.

7.003   Subjectively inefficient thinking

Those affected complain that they are unable to think clearly, that their brain is working less efficiently than their normal. They are unable to reach decisions easily, even about simple matters, because they cannot maintain the necessary elements of information in consciousness at the same time. It is thus the internal equivalent of loss of concentration. Thoughts are muddled and tend to go round and round in aimless circles. This complaint is subjective, and may be in contrast to the clear and efficient way in which subjects describe the symptom. Only the subjective complaint is rated. However, the following three criteria must always apply: the experience is unpleasant, it does not respond to subjects' voluntary attempts to end it, and it is out of proportion to the difficulties of the problems being considered. In order to meet the severity criterion for a rating of (3), there should either be extreme muddling or marked subjective slowing.

Some subjects may complain that their thought processes have always been muddled, throughout their lives. This should be rated (7).

Differentiation from other symptoms:

There may be several reasons for the symptom, including worrying, inefficiency of thinking, distractibility, anxiety, poor concentration, etc. The rating should be made on the basis of whether the symptom is present, not on what its cause is thought to be.

If thought insertion, commentary, withdrawal or broadcast (items **18.005 - 18.011**) are present, or other psychotic experiences or explanations or thought or speech disorder that make the rating difficult, rate (5).

7.004   Loss of Interests

There is a definite recent diminution in the Respondent's interests, either some interests have been dropped, or the intensity of interest has decreased. Everyone has interests of some sort, but the extent of any diminution must be measured in the context of the range and depth of their usual activities. Take into account everyday vocational and domestic activities as well as leisure pursuits, keeping well-informed, taking an interest in clothes, food and appearance, keeping up to date with the news, etc. Inevitably, those with the most intense and varied interests initially will have most room to lose interest and those who have never taken a great interest in things will not have much to lose. An appreciable diminution in the general level of interests is rated (2); almost complete loss is rated (3).

7.005   Subjective Feeling of Retardation

Those afflicted feel as though they are moving markedly more slowly than usual, that they walk as though they were older than their age. One described it as 'like walking in treacle'. Speech may also seem to be slowed. When very severe there is a subjective feeling of being hardly able to move or speak at all. Objective slowness is likely to be observed in such a case (items **22.002 - 22.007**). Item **7.005**, however, is concerned only with the subjectively described experience.

If present on and off for two years or more, consider rating the checklist on dysthymia.

7.006   Loss of Energy (Drive)

Loss of energy is expressed in terms of feeling weak, floppy, of having lost one's get-up-and go, one's vigor. Initiating a task, whether physical or mental, seems difficult, even impossible. Everything seems too much trouble.

Differentiation from other symptoms:

The symptom may underlie others, such as tedium vitae (item **6.012**), loss of concentration or interests (items **7.002** and **7.004**), and a feeling of inability to cope with everyday tasks (item **7.007**), but these are defined more in terms of the accompanying content. Anergia is a relatively 'basic' symptom that does not depend on context or content for its definition.

If present on and off for two years or more, consider rating the checklist on dysthymia.

7.007 Feeling of being overwhelmed by everyday tasks

This may arise from lack of energy (item **7.006**) or as a consequence of apathy and subjective retardation (item **7.005**), often aggravated by negative self-attitudes. It consists of a tendency to shy away mentally from the prospect of any constructive activity. Even the contemplation of tasks is painful, out of proportion to the mental and physical effort required, and subjectively very difficult to overcome. If present on and off for two years or more, consider rating the checklist on dysthymia.

7.008 Dates of PERIOD/S of Section 7 symptoms

8   Bodily functions

GENERAL POINTS ABOUT ITEMS 8.001 - 8.008, APPETITE AND WEIGHT

If R is in an episode of disorder it will usually be necessary to rate Section 8 items for that period.

It should be kept in mind that symptoms in Section 8 are grouped together for convenience. It will often be necessary to take them out of order, for example when rating an affective episode or eating disorder. Some rating scales specifically require a decision as to whether the symptom is associated with a depressive episode.

However, all can (and in population surveys do) occur without being part of any specific mental or physical disorder. The period to be rated is specified for some items; if R is not in episode, rate the others for the past month (PS check).

Weight problems related to physical disorders are rated using the etiology option.

8.001 - 8.004   Weight, height and change since adolescence

To obtain a baseline in young patients or those who have been persistently under or overweight, estimate postpubertal weight (e.g. aged before 20). In cases of prepubertal-onset anorexia nervosa, estimate change from weight at the onset of the condition.

8.005   Poor Appetite or increased appetite

Food and the thought of food is not attractive even when a meal is due. Food has lost its savor - 'it is like eating cardboard'. It may take a great effort to go through the motions of chewing and swallowing. Weight may not be lost, if intake is maintained as an act of deliberate policy. Increased appetite, if almost daily should be rated (4,) or (5) if for longer than 2 weeks. Patients with anorexia nervosa may or may not show poor appetite, regardless of their avoidance of food.

8.006   Weight Loss or Gain
8.007

In order for weight loss or gain to be rated (1) or (2), it must be the result of a change in appetite. If there is a possibility of Anorexia or Bulimia Nervosa use the information in Section 9. Rate maximum weight change during period even if original appetite and weight has been restored through recovery.

Weight loss secondary to a physical condition should be rated using the etiology option.

8.008   Weight problem

This general probe allows an exploration of the nature of any weight problem that has not been resolved so far.

8.009 - 8.012   General points about sleep problems

It should be possible to rate these items by obtaining an overall account of sleeping patterns during the period. Ratings may be difficult to make in people who work nights, or varying shifts like aircrews. In such cases, make the rating only if there is clear evidence of disturbance; i.e. rate a departure from the usual diurnal rhythm rather than time of day.

Sleep problems related to physical disorders or external physical causes (medication, psychoactive substance use etc.) are rated using the etiology option.

8.013   Middle Insomnia

Middle insomnia includes periods of wakefulness between an initial and a final period of sleep.

8.014   Early Waking

This refers to the time of waking after the final period of sleep during the night i.e. the subject should not sleep again afterwards. Take R's occupation into account; i.e. rate a departure from the usual diurnal rhythm rather than time of day.

Differentiation from other symptoms:

If the subject does fall asleep again after 'early waking', rate middle insomnia (item **8.013**).

The rating should be made on the basis of a change from the usual pattern. Consider the possibility that some people are characteristically early risers. Early rising may derive from the demands of early working hours and may persist for years after retirement or job change.

Waking early and refreshed in an episode of mania should not be rated here, but at item **10.013**.

8.015   Disturbance of Sleep-Wake Cycle

In the extreme form there may be day-night reversal - the subject may potter about all night and sleep during the day. Usually however, it involves staying awake until well into the small hours followed by sleep, e.g. from 5 a.m. to 1 p.m. It is sometimes seen in unemployed people, and may be a feature of social peculiarity in schizophrenia and Asperger syndrome. If an adaptation to permanent night shift work, it should be excluded.

8.016   Hypersomnia

Sleeping at least two hours longer than usual. There must be a definite change from R's usual pattern. Irresistible sleepiness is usually associated, as is a period of 'sleep drunkenness' after waking. A rating of (2) means that the condition has lasted more or less daily for a month or more.

Differentiation from other symptoms:

Sleepiness alone would not usually be sufficient for a rating, unless exceptionally severe and not due to poor sleep at night. Making up by daytime sleep for hours lost at night is also not included. There should usually be at least two hours of sleep or associated irresistible sleepiness.

Pathological fatigue is rated at items **2.040, 2.041, 2.042, and 3.007**.

Narcolepsy should be rated using the etiology option. Associated features include: cataplexy, sleep paralysis, hypnagogic hallucinations, sleep apnea (nocturnal breath cessation, intermittent snorting sounds).

8.017   Disturbing Dreams or Nightmares

This item is rated on the basis of the distress caused by the nightmares, but this is usually related to frequency. Many people have occasional frightening dreams, involving threats to survival, security or self-esteem, from which they may wake up feeling frightened, followed by relief, as full consciousness dawns. Nightmares commonly occur in the second half of the night and the subject is quickly oriented after waking up. Differentiate from night terrors. If the Respondent is distressed by nightmares several times in a fortnight, rate (1). If several times in a week, rate (2).

8.018   Sleep Terrors

Respondents with this symptom report (or have been informed by reliable observers that they) repeatedly wake from sleep in terror, with intense autonomic anxiety and bodily motility. They may rush out of bed screaming, and are often disoriented for 1 to 10 minutes and at risk of injury. For a time they are unresponsive even to familiar others. There is a failure to recall events that preceded the waking up.

8.019   Sleepwalking

This rating must be based on information from others than the Respondent. The symptom usually occurs during the first third of the sleep period and lasts between 1 and 10 minutes. Those affected rise from bed and walk about for periods up to 30 minutes. During this time they have a blank face, are unresponsive to others who try to wake them. After waking, they have amnesia for the episode and may briefly be confused, but there is no persistent impairment. There are repeated episodes.

8.024 Sexual dysfunction

To make this rating, it is required that the Respondent normally has some sexual interest and that this has been lost during the period evaluated. The symptom should be rated on the basis of the subject's level of interest, not only on overt sexual activity. People without a partner may still be aware of a diminution of responsiveness towards the preferred sex, a responsiveness that need not involve any serious sexual fantasy. Where the subject does have a partner, it is usually easier to make the rating on the basis of attitude towards actual sexual activity. The ratings are self explanatory.

If any physical condition accounts for recent loss of libido, use the etiology option.

8.025 Loss of libido associated with depression

Item **8.025** allows any association with depressed mood to be rated.

8.026 Intercourse unpleasant

This item is a general probe for problems connected with intercourse. An associated schedule will be prepared by WHO to cover other aspects of sexual dysfunction.

9 Eating disorders

GENERAL POINTS ABOUT SECTION 9

Items in this Section are concerned with problems connected with weight, preoccupation with body shape, and undereating and overeating. The period covered is the year before interview, and an earlier episode can be rated if necessary for research purposes.

All respondents who are underweight, or who have been unduly concerned with weight and shape during the year, but not clearly related to physical or nutritional disorders, should be considered. (Weight at the time of interview may not reflect changes that have occurred during the year).

The technical definition of 'underweight' is 15% below weight for age and height.

9.001 Dread of Being or Becoming Fat

This is an introductory probe for Anorexia and also for Bulimia. The main characteristic is a fear or severe worry about being or becoming fat or overweight that persists as an intrusive over-valued idea. Include a feeling of being too fat or a fear of gaining weight at a time when underweight.

9.002 Earlier episode of undereating

Decide at this point whether a previous episode of Anorexia should be rated for research or other particular purposes. If so, it can be rated at the same time as PY or after it. The dates are recorded at item **9.019**. Enter 1 if there has been one or more previous episode.

9.003 Irresistible and persistent craving for food

This is a further probe for bulimia.

9.004 Earlier episode of overeating

Decide at this point whether a previous episode of Bulimia should be rated for research or other particular purposes. If so, it can be rated at the same time as PY or after it. The dates are recorded at item **9.020**. Enter 1 if there has been one or more previous episode.

9.005 Interference due to appetite problems

This item relates to the ability to carry out normal activities and roles. This tends to be progressively impaired as anorexia or bulimia persist. Some people are affected at a relatively early stage, others not until later. There may be a precipitate collapse of function. Rate actual performance, as indicated in the scale. (Another opportunity to rate this item, in the context of other symptoms, is provided at item **13.010**. The Section 13 rating will overwrite **9.005**.)

CUT-OFF POINT

Always continue below the cut-off point if there is any reason to suppose that any of the remaining Section 9 items are present.

9.006   Undue preoccupation with bodily shape

This item allows further probing as to whether any of the body image problems, and consequent imposition of a low weight threshold, that underlie Anorexia and Bulimia Nervosa, are present. The symptom is an intense over-valued idea.

9.007   Imposes low weight threshold

The subject maintains body weight at least 15% below the expected normal weight

9.008   Avoidance of Fattening Foods

Rate any major alteration in diet designed to lower weight. This includes avoidance of high calorie foods and the severe restriction of total food intake. Exclude alteration in intake as part of normal dieting.

9.009   Action to lose weight through self restriction

The subject induces weight loss by self-medication with appetite suppressants.

9.010   Action to lose weight through purgation

The subject induces weight loss by self-induced purging using laxatives. Excessive exercise and taking diuretics are other methods employed by the subject for weight loss.

9.011   Prepubertal onset of anorexia

The sequence of pubertal events is delayed or arrested and growth ceases. In girls the breasts do not develop and there is a primary amenorrhea. With recovery there is a delayed menarche. In boys the genitals remain juvenile unless there is recovery.

9.012   Change in sexual functioning

9.013   Binge Eating

Rate recurring cravings for food that are not resisted. Large quantities of food are consumed in a short space of time, with loss of control.

9.014 Dread of getting fat in spite of craving

This is this same symptom as **9.001** but in a context of overeating with loss of control. Make a separate rating.

9.015 Actions to correct binging by purgation

After binging, the subject attempts to counteract the fattening effects of food by self-medication with laxatives.

9.016 Restrictive actions to correct binging

After binging, the subject attempts to counteract the fattening effects of food by fasting, starvation or excessive exercise.

9.017 Age present episode of anorexia started

9.018 Age present episode of bulimia started

9.019 Age at first onset of anorexia

9.020 Age at first onset of bulimia

9.021 Dates of previous episode of anorexia

9.022 Dates of previous episode of bulimia

9.023 Relation of Bulimia to Anorexia

Rate here the relationship of bulimia to anorexia.

9.024 Dates of PERIOD/S rated at Section 9
9.025

9.026 Interference with activities due to Section 9 symptoms

Rate the degree of interference with normal everyday activities due to presence of Section 9 symptoms.

10 Expansive mood and ideation

GENERAL POINTS ABOUT SECTION 10

To comply with the diagnostic requirements of ICD-10 and DSM-IV for mania and hypomania, expansive or irritable mood must be rated for severity, because the number of required manic symptoms differ depending on the quality of the mood. Irritability (**3.009**) should be checked and rated independently, not being fully identical with irritable mood.

The hypomanic/manic symptoms (**10.004 - 10.015**) also must be rated by severity to be able to discern between ICD-10 hypomania and mania, the duration having been rated at item **10.003**. In ICD-10, the diagnostic criteria are different for hypomania and mania, with mild to moderate symptoms for hypomania, leading to only some interference with functioning, and more severe symptoms for mania with severe interference.

Some of the course items in Section 6 (**6.030 - 6.036**), apply also to Section 10. They must always be considered, and if necessary re-rated, before leaving the Section. The dates of previous episodes should also be rated if R is in a relapse episode.

Dysthymia is rated at items **6.044 - 6.061**. Cyclothymia requires ratings on items **10.019 - 10.050** which are called 'hypomania' and are often (but not necessarily) mixed with dysthymic symptoms.

10.001 Expansive (elevated) mood

The subject is euphoric or elated most of the time. 'Most of the time' is interpreted to include frequent brief periods of elation if part of 'rapid cycling'. The mood often has an infectious quality, and in extreme cases those affected may be in a state of exaltation. The mood is out of proportion to the subject's circumstances, which may indeed be uncertain if not downright depressing. Transient high spirits concordant with circumstances should therefore not be included. There is usually an element of excitement, irritability (rate predominantly irritable mood at **10.002**) or suspicion, which the patient may recognize as disturbing or unhealthy. Occasionally the symptom may be more transient but very frequently repeated - it should then still be rated as present.

An element of judgement is required for this rating since respondents sometimes do not recognize their mood as having been expansive once it is past, but may simply describe themselves as having been cheerful or in ordinary good spirits. Take care not to miss the symptom because of this.

10.002 Irritable mood

Irritable, irascible erethism or excitability. A pervasive mood of angry impatience, hair splitting querulance, hasty temper, and easily aroused aggressiveness.

10.003 Duration of expansive or irritable mood

Duration is rated at this item. Present but less than 4 days rate 1; at least 4 days rate 2; at least one week rate 3; more than 2 months rate 4; hospital admission required rate 5 irrespective of duration.

10.004 Pressing and racing thoughts

This symptom is the subjective aspect of flight of ideas. Images and ideas flash through the mind, each suggesting others, at a fast rate. If the state persists over a period covering at least 4 days, it should be rated (1). More persistent forms are rated according to the schedule guidelines.

10.005 Overtalkativeness

Respondents may sense a pressure to keep talking but, more often, it is others who notice an abnormality. Speech is fluent, rapid and loud. There may be overcircumstantiality and shifts of topic, but conversation can be conducted with wit. It may be possible to rate this item from self-description, but respondents may also report the comments of others at the time which corroborate their account.

10.006 Distractibility

This is the external equivalent of flight of ideas, in the sense that it reflects intrusions from sources in the environment. The flow of thought is disrupted by the attachment of the respondent's attention to chance aspects of the surroundings.

10.007 Self-reported overactivity

Overactivity is expressed in motor behavior as well as speech and ideation. Those affected have tremendous energy, are far more active than usual, their movements are rapid and they do not need so much sleep as usual. Substantiation of the rating may be obtained by asking about the responses of their neighbors, who may have complained bitterly e.g. about loud music played late at night.

10.008 Sharpened thinking

The ability of those affected to concentrate to concentrate, solve problems be creative etc. seems unequivocally well beyond the ordinary mode. However they do not necessarily construe this increased mental facility as connoting superior or extraordinary intelligence when compared to others. This symptom is often accompanied by inflated self-esteem but exaggerated self-esteem is rated separately in item **10.010**.

10.009 Overly entertaining talk

This symptom is different from overtalkativeness (rated in item **10.005**) but usually is associated with it. Those affected can persistently make numerous and witty remarks or reports and rhyming, punning and jovial conversation which is often inappropriate.

10.010 Exaggerated self-esteem

Those affected may feel that they are superbly healthy, have exceptionally high intelligence or extraordinary abilities.

The borderline between this symptom and 'grandiose delusions' (items **10.016 / 19.029, 10.017 / 19.030**) is difficult to draw, except that grandiose ideas are simply exaggerations of the subjects' normal state (e.g. they may actually be capable and intelligent or have some particular ability), whereas delusions involve an identification or an assertion that is demonstrably false (e.g. that the Respondent is a king or invented the atom-bomb). In either case, however, insight tends to be lacking.

10.011 Overoptimism

Unduly optimistic view of the past and future. Include retrospective falsification and exaggeration of past achievements that are neither facetious "tall-tales" nor delusional convictions (item **10.016**). Also include a sense of luckiness not based on respondents perceived capabilities.

10.012 Actions based on expansive mood

The cognitive component of expansive mood may be translated into action: gambling, inappropriate gifts to charity, reckless driving, unaccustomed drunkenness, spending sprees. Such actions may or may not be socially embarrassing (item **10.014**). Increased libido is rated at item **10.015**. In order to obtain an account, it may be useful to remind the respondent of material recorded in the case records. Indiscreet behavior should only be rated here if it is clearly based on grandiose ideas and expansive mood.

10.013 Decreased need for sleep

This is another reflection of overactivity although not a universal one; some of those affected exhaust themselves in their daytime activities. Others go to bed in the small hours, wake early, feeling refreshed after a short sleep, and are eager to begin another overactive day.

10.014 Socially embarrassing behavior

Loss of normal social inhibitions may lead to unwise and embarrassing behavior, including overfamiliarity, quarrels and foolish actions that are both out of character and inappropriate to the circumstances at the time.

10.015   Increased sexual drive or activity

The symptom may be expressed in increased sexual activity with the usual partner, or in increased flirtatiousness, or in sexual indiscretions.

10.016 - 10.017   Expansive delusions

These items are repeated in Part II of SCAN at items **19.029** and **19.030**. Hallucinations in affective psychoses are rated at **6.021 / 17.010 / 17.011** and this item should be re-checked. If ratings are made in Section 10, the computer program allocates them to their equivalents in Part II. If both sets of items are rated, the Part II items are given preference. It should be noted that other relevant psychological and behavioral abnormalities are rated only in Part II, for example, increased motor activity at **22.015 - 22.018** and **22.020**. If there is any doubt as to whether to proceed to Part II, always do so.

10.018   Age at first onset of Section 10 symptoms

This item provides an opportunity to check the entry made at **1.016**.

10.019   Mixed episodes during the episode of illness

A mixed episode is characterized by either a mixture or a rapid alternation of hypomanic or manic with depressive symptoms. Rate 3 if the current episode is mixed.

10.020   Date of PE or RE

10.022 - 10.027   Dates of earlier PERIODS of expansive mood

Instructions for dating earlier periods are provided in Section 6 (**6.038** to **6.043**). Rate quality of remissions between episodes at **1.018**.

10.028   Interference with activities due to Section 10 symptoms

Rate the degree of interference with subject's normal everyday activities because of Section 10 symptoms.

10.029   Organic cause of Section 10 symptoms

Rating of phenomenology should in general be made without consideration of etiology. The etiology option allows individual items to be separately rated for an etiological attribution.

Item **10.029** allows a simple rating of whether an 'organic' cause is present, whether or not it can be specified in terms of an ICD-10 class. Four general rules are used to make such attributions of cause:

(a) Evidence of cerebral disorder, damage or dysfunction, whether direct or via non-cerebral disorder or toxicity.

(b) A temporal relationship between the development of the disease and the onset of the symptoms in Section 10; such as onset of symptoms within 3 months (before or after) the presumed cause.

(c) Recovery or improvement after removal of the cause.

(d) No other obvious cause.

If these criteria are met for expansive symptoms, rate (1). Use (8) if uncertain. The default rating is (0).

10.030 ICD Code for Organic cause of Section 10 symptoms

Anti-depressive drugs, steroids, endocrine disorders such as hyper- and hypo-thyroidism and hyper- or hypo-adrenocorticalism, and infectious diseases, may be associated with manic symptoms. The letter identifying the ICD-10 chapter, and up to three digits, should be entered at item **10.030**. A list of ICD-10 categories is provided in the Appendix.

If any psychoactive substances rated in Section 12 are thought to cause manic symptoms, make the causal attributions in Section 12.

10.031 - 10.050 Checklist: cyclothymia and persistent hypomania

A period of at least 2 years of instability of mood, involving periods of hypomania or of hypomania with dysthymia, with or without periods of normal mood.

The symptoms of dysthymia have been rated at items **6.044 - 6.061**. Those of persistent hypomania are listed at **10.031 - 10.050**. Most are rated elsewhere in Part I of SCAN. They are identified by a line reading, 'If > 2 years consider cyclothymia'. Only the ratings of the hypomanic component should be made at this Checklist.

Since it will often not be clear, before the interview begins, whether hypomanic symptoms have lasted for more than 2 years and whether the other course criteria apply, the appropriate strategy is to make general enquiries about the course at the beginning of Section 10 to supplement those already made for Dysthymia. If R is clearly in an episode of major depression or mania it is not necessary to complete either Checklist, except for research purposes. (The status of the disorders will be clarified by co-morbidity studies).

11 Use of alcohol

GENERAL POINTS ABOUT SECTION 11

The items in Sections 11 and 12 follow a similar pattern. The first item provides an opportunity to skip out of the Section. Items on quantity and frequency come next, followed by sufficient above cut-off items to allow a decision as to whether a disorder is present. Below cut-off items reflect more serious problems. There is a final subsection concerned with dating the onset and offset of dependency and harm 'syndromes'. If the respondent is not a life time abstainer, all subsequent questions should be asked in sections 11 and 12, except where skip outs are indicated.

11.001 Lifetime abstention from alcohol

The first question needs to be asked in a way that takes into account what is already known about R and R's culture. If necessary, rephrase it more appropriately, using words like "alcoholic beverages" or "drinks with alcohol" to clarify the meaning of the question. The item provides an opportunity to skip out of the Section if there has been no, or virtually no, use of alcohol at any time. It is followed by a set of probes, to be amplified or varied at the interviewer's judgement, designed to obtain an account of the pattern and effects of R's use of alcohol. This forms the basis for the rest of the Section. It is not necessary to repeat questions later if the answers have already been obtained in this introductory description.

11.002 Frequency of drinking, past year

Enter R's estimate of frequency of drinking during the past year. Quantity is not taken into account. If R has had extended periods of abstinence during past year or lifetime before, code frequency of drinking during heaviest period.

11.003 Estimated usual daily alcohol (PY and LB)

This question attempts to estimate the usual amount of ethanol taken on an average (typical or usual) day when R drinks. The method used in SCAN is to ask which types of alcoholic drink R typically takes (wine, beer, spirits, or a combination of these), what volume is typically consumed (a pint, a glass, etc.) and how much alcohol the glass or container contains. This information can most practically be obtained by showing R a chart, with a range of glasses containing the alcoholic beverages typically available in that community, in "standard drink" format. A standard drink is the amount of ethanol contained in standard glasses of beer, wine, fortified wine such as sherry, and spirits. In most countries these amounts are roughly equivalent and range between 8 and 14 grams of ethanol. In countries where there is great variability in the amounts consumed on a given occasion, or if R drinks infrequently in variable amounts, record an average or median between the high and low amounts mentioned. The number of standard drinks is therefore calculated, not on the amount of alcohol averaged over all days in the year, but over the days when R drinks. Frequency of drinking is recorded elsewhere.

11.004 Heavier daily alcohol (PY and LB)

This item is designed to measure drinking during periods of "heavier" or maximum alcohol consumption such as binges, festivals, weekends, and holidays. If the amount entered for the usual amount is the same, enter it again. Probe for LB as well as PY.

11.005 Frequency of heavier daily alcohol (PY and LB)

If the heavier use is more than the usual or average quantity taken when R drinks, estimate an approximate frequency of the heavier drinking. If heavy use is about equal to the usual daily intake of alcohol, enter the same code.

11.006 Most recent drink

Information about R's most recent alcohol use can be useful for a variety of reasons. If R has been drinking within the past 24 hours, the acute effects of alcohol, "hangover" effects or withdrawal symptoms may influence the validity and reliability of information provided during the SCAN interview. Whenever possible, do not interview patients during periods of intoxication or withdrawal.

11.007 Subjective need for alcohol (PY and LB)

This aspect of alcohol dependence is manifested by a persistent preoccupation with alcohol and drinking. R feels uneasy at times or in places where alcohol is not available. Often this symptom is identified as a craving: (an unbearable and intensive desire to drink or taste alcohol, which can arise in response to the sight, smell or taste of it or of stimuli that have been associated with drinking in the past). It is important to distinguish this strong subjective need for alcohol from merely being thirsty for a drink, as in temperate climates where beer, palm wine or pulque are consumed as a thirst quencher. Rate (1) if R reports persistent thoughts but not a strong desire or craving. Rate (2) if there is a strong and intrusive preoccupation.

11.008 Impaired capacity to abstain/cut drinking (PY and LB)

R expresses a desire to stop drinking, but reports that repeated attempts have been unsuccessful. Typically these attempts include rules and other stratagems to avoid alcohol entirely or to limit the frequency of drinking. Resumption of heavy drinking after seeking professional help for a drinking problem, or joining a mutual help group such as Alcoholics Anonymous, would be evidence of lack of success. Rate 1 if R has voluntarily abstained or effectively controlled drinking for a month or more. Rate 2 if R has failed to abstain for a month or more. Also rate 2 if R has only been able to control drinking with the help of treatment, mutual-help groups (e.g. Alcoholics Anonymous) or removal to a controlled environment (e.g. prison).

11.009　Impaired capacity to control drinking once started (PY and LB)

The subject is aware (or can be made aware) of an impaired capacity to control the amount of alcohol taken or the ability to terminate use. This impaired control includes inability to prevent spontaneous onset of drinking bouts as well as failure to stop drinking before intoxication develops. This behavior should be distinguished from situations in which the subject's control over the onset or amount of drinking is strongly affected by social or cultural factors, such as drinking that may occur during celebrations and festive occasions. One way to judge the degree of impaired control is to determine whether R has made repeated attempts to limit the quantity of drinking, using such tactics as making rules or imposing limits on access to alcohol. The more these attempts have failed, the more the subject manifests impaired control. Code 3 only if there is evidence of severely impaired control, such as binges. A binge is defined as a period of relatively continuous drinking and intoxication lasting more than one day. It is often indicative of impaired control, especially when social influences or cultural factors (e.g., "fiesta drinking") are not responsible for maintaining the binge.

> **NOTE:　The following items (11.010, 11.011, 11.019, and 11.023) refer to harm caused by alcohol. For harm to be rated the nature of harm should be clearly identifiable and must occur for month at a stretch or repeatedly over a year.**

11.010　Social problems due to drinking (PY and LB)

Alcohol use can be associated with a wide variety of social consequences that result from the direct effects of intoxication (e.g. absence from school or intoxication at work), the indirect effects of intoxication (criticism by employer or spouse) or the cumulative effects of heavy drinking (e.g. financial problems, marital discord). The social consequences of alcohol are sometimes affected by the drinker's age, gender and culture. In extreme situations (e.g. severe criticism of moderate drinking by a total abstainer), these mitigating factors should be taken into account in rating the severity of problems due to drinking. Social problems should be rated only when they are the result of impaired judgement or dysfunctional behavior that are a direct consequence of alcohol use.

11.011　Legal problems due to drinking (PY and LB)

Drinking can be the cause of legal problems of varying severity, either directly related to drinking (e.g. being arrested for drunk-driving, being sued for physical violence toward a family member under the influence of alcohol, being put in jail for public drunkenness) or indirectly related to drinking (e.g. being sued for inability to pay debts because of drinking expenses, having legal action taken for divorce or inability to fulfill child support obligations). Rate legal problems when they are a result of impaired judgement or dysfunctional behavior that are a direct consequence of alcohol use.

11.012 Persistent drinking after social and/or legal harm (PY and LB)

The key aspect of this symptom is the persistence of drinking in spite of knowledge of social harm, such as loss of employment or legal problems. If R stopped drinking, cut down on the frequency or amount of alcohol use, or otherwise made successful efforts to control drinking and avoid future problems, then score this question as 0 (No). If these changes were only temporary, after which the subject returned to the same pattern of high risk drinking, score 1 (Yes). If R does not realize or is not aware that harm is due to alcohol, rate 0.

11.013 Failure to fulfill major role obligations (PY and LB)

A common symptom of dependence is the inability to fulfill major role obligations because of drinking or intoxication. If there is evidence that drinking is only incidental to lack of role performance, code this item zero. Obligations should be culturally appropriate - if the subject's culture considers fiesta drinking appropriate male behavior during carnival time, do not necessarily code binge drinking as a neglect of work or family obligations, unless such drinking goes beyond common custom.

11.014 Risk taking behavior with alcohol (PY and LB).

The risk of getting hurt or of hurting others should be rated according to the severity of risk and whether it involves self or others. Take into account R's degree of tolerance and the kinds of risk most common in the respondent's environment. The rating should be made on assessment of risk, not simply of quantity of alcohol. For example, does R know the (low) limits within which he or she can drink and drive safely and act within them? Rate 1 if there has been risk-taking behavior during the period. Rate 2 if harm has actually occurred to self or others because of drinking.

CUT-OFF POINT

The threshold for cut-off has deliberately been set low since there are no empirical data on which to base it. This carries a danger that some respondents will be offended by what they see as unnecessary and intrusive questioning. The interviewer should take this into account in subsequent questioning.

11.015 Salience of drink-related activities (PY and LB)

A characteristic symptom is that drinking is given a higher priority than other activities, in spite of its negative consequences. There is a progressive neglect of alternative pleasures or interests in favor of alcohol use. There is a diminished responsiveness of the individual to the normal processes of informal social control. Drinking or alcohol intoxication interferes with R's ability to conform to tacit social rules governing activities, such as keeping appointments, caring for children, that are typically expected by the drinker's reference group.

11.016 Time involved in drink-related activities (PY and LB)

The amount of time or effort devoted to obtaining, using or recovering from alcohol use is a symptom of the degree of dependence. If R spends a great deal of time in drinking-related activities, such as a month or more of daily or continuous involvement, rate (2). If less time is spent on alcohol use, rate (1). This needs to be distinguished from cases where "time spent drinking" is conditioned by cultural expectations and contexts. In some cultures, adult males may spend a considerable amount of time in a cafe, tavern or public house, even though their alcohol consumption is not excessive. Time spent drinking is symptomatic only when it displaces other activities or obligations in order to permit more time for alcohol consumption as the primary end in itself.

11.017 Narrowing of drinking pattern (PY and LB)

Narrowing refers to the tendency of alcohol use to become progressively stereotyped around a prescribed routine of customs and rituals. Narrowing is characterized by increased facility of performance; accustomed doses; and lack of variation in time, place or manner of drinking. Rate (0) if drinking is not associated with prescribed or habitual customs or rituals, or if there is a stereotyped pattern of only light or moderate drinking. Rate (1) if there is some regularity to the heavy drinking pattern. Rate (2) if the pattern is fixed with regard to time, place or manner of use, and R finds it very difficult to deviate from it.

11.018 Tolerance to alcohol (PY and LB)

Tolerance may be physical, behavioral or psychological. In relation to earlier phases of R's drinking history, increased doses of alcohol are required to achieve effects originally produced by lower doses and/or diminished effects are achieved by doses used at an earlier time. A clear example would be the consumption of amounts that would have seriously impaired or even proved lethal on previous occasions. Rate (0) if no tolerance is suggested. Rate (1) if there is some tolerance but R still experiences impairment at high doses. Rate (2) if marked tolerance is suggested by little or no apparent impairment even at high blood alcohol concentrations.

Reversed tolerance is rated (3). This is the development of sensitivity to doses of alcohol that formerly would have been tolerated without intoxicating effects. It can occur after cutting down on drinking or during the normal aging process.

11.019 Psychological and Mental health problems due to drinking (PY and LB)

Alcohol use is associated with a wide variety of psychological and mental health problems that result from the direct effects of intoxication (e.g. aggressive behavior), the sequelae of intoxication (e.g. depression, delusional symptoms) or the cumulative effects of heavy drinking (e.g. insomnia, depression, paranoid thinking). The attribution of cause is made in this item. If more than one type of symptom is caused (for example, hallucinations and depression) choose the most severe. The scale is in order of severity of type of symptom, with 9 the most severe.

The severity of the mental symptoms themselves is not rated here but in the relevant Sections of PSE10. Exclude social problems and physical health problems rated at items **11.010** and **11.023** as well as neglect of obligations and time lost due to drinking rated in **11.013** and **11.016**. Exclude physiological effects of intoxication and withdrawal.

The presence and severity of psychiatric symptoms is rated in detail throughout SCAN, and the relevant sections should be considered before rating this item. The purpose of the item is to specify whether alcohol is the cause of the most severe type of symptom present. A clinical judgement should be based on all the information available, not just the answers to the probes. In the case of psychotic symptoms (e.g. alcoholic hallucinosis) an attribution of cause should only be made if there is no or only minor clouding; onset is typically within 48 hours but not later than two weeks after the last drink. To be rated here, any psychotic symptoms should persist for at least 48 hours but not more than 6 months. Rate the form of cognitive impairment of various kinds due to alcohol, at items **21.112, 21.116, 21.119** and **21.120**. Mental health problems due to alcohol may also be rated in Sections 13 and 20.

11.020 Onset of alcohol-induced mental health problems

The purpose of this item is to differentiate where possible between psychiatric problems that are associated with intoxication, alcohol withdrawal, or neither. This is done by indicating the circumstances under which symptoms directly attributed to alcohol had their onset.

11.021 Interference due to alcohol-induced symptoms (PY and LB)

Rate the degree of interference resulting from the worst mental health symptoms coded in item **11.019**. Exclude social problems and physical health problems rated at items **11.010** and **11.023** as well as neglect of obligations and time lost due to drinking rated in **11.013** and **11.016**. Exclude physiological effects of intoxication and withdrawal.

11.022 Persistent drinking after mental harm (PY and LB)

The key aspect of this symptom is the persistence of drinking in spite of knowledge of mental harm, such as depressive symptoms or hallucinations. If R stopped drinking, cut down on the frequency or amount of alcohol use, or made other successful efforts to control drinking and avoid future problems, then score this question as 0 (No). If these changes were only temporary, after which the subject returned to the same pattern of high risk drinking, score 1 (Yes). If R does not realize or is not aware that harm is due to alcohol, rate 0.

11.023 Physical health problems due to drinking (PY and LB)

Alcohol use can be associated with a wide variety of health problems such as liver disease, pancreatitis, duodenal ulcer, peripheral neuropathy, and traumatic injury. Rate severity of health problems according to the degree of functional disability reported by respondent: (1) refers to mild physical illness, or functional disability; (2) refers to physical illness of moderate severity. Rate (3) if R's alcohol-related problems are life threatening.

Use the Clinical History Schedule to record the ICD-10 categories of any physical illness due to alcohol. If memory impairment rate **11.019** and Section 21.

11.024 Persistent drinking after physical harm (PY and LB)

The key aspect in rating this symptom of alcohol dependence is the persistence of drinking in spite of knowledge of physical harm, such as liver disease or traumatic injury. If R stopped drinking, cut down on the frequency or amount of alcohol use, or otherwise made successful efforts to control drinking and avoid future problems, then score this question as 0 (No). If these changes were only temporary, after which R returned to the same pattern of high risk drinking, score 1 (Yes). If R does not realize or is not aware that harm is due to alcohol, rate 0.

11.025 Alcohol withdrawal problems (PY and LB)

Check for tachycardia or hypertension, sweating, insomnia, tactile or visual perceptual abnormalities, nausea, diarrhea, headache, tremor, weakness, restlessness, and autonomic anxiety. Recall somatic and neurotic symptoms rated in earlier sections. Did any of these start hours after withdrawal or cutting down, following a period of heavy drinking? If present at examination, include the past year. Delirium with or without fits is rated 3 and attributed to alcohol at **21.119 / 21.120**.

These problems do not necessarily occur together and vary in degree of severity. They tend to occur after repeated, and usually prolonged and/or high-dose use of ethanol. In addition to physical withdrawal symptoms, psychological disturbances (e.g. anxiety, depression) and sleep disturbance are also common features. While continued ethanol use may lead to the manifestation of mild withdrawal symptoms even on the basis of brief periods of abstinence (e.g. after a typical night of sleep), some persistent drinkers may have never had a long enough period of abstinence to permit withdrawal to occur. It is therefore important to ask if R ever had a period of abstinence longer than several days. Rate degree of withdrawal effects according to the frequency and severity of effects (scale points 0-2). If convulsions and delirium occur as withdrawal effects, rate (3). If delirium or fits are toxic effects, rate at item **11.031**. All cognitive problems should also be rated in Section 21.

11.026 Drinking to relieve or avoid withdrawal (PY and LB)

R uses alcohol with the intention of relieving or avoiding withdrawal symptoms and with an awareness that this strategy is effective. Morning drinking to relieve nausea or the 'shakes' is the most common behavior signalling manifestation of relief drinking. Use of alcohol to relieve hangovers should not be coded as relief drinking unless the hangovers are part of withdrawal syndrome.

NB: **For rating acute toxic effects of alcohol ensure that the symptoms or signs are not better accounted for by another medical disorder unrelated to alcohol use or by another mental or behavioral disorder.**

11.027 Pathological / Idiosyncratic reaction to alcohol (PY and LB)

Alcohol use is sometimes associated with pathological and/or idiosyncratic reactions that may or may not be caused by the pharmacological effects of ethanol. Idiosyncratic reactions consist of untypically aggressive or violent behavior, within minutes to an hour or so after drinking, with no evidence of physical intoxication to account for it. It is often followed by amnesia for the occasion.

If there is evidence of intoxication being associated with inappropriate social behavior (e.g. sexual harassment or sexual disinhibition) or aggressive behavior, code 2, 3 or 4, as appropriate, but only when behavior is manifested during intoxication. If behavior also occurs when subject is not drinking, do not code as an alcohol reaction.

11.028 Acute toxic effects of alcohol, uncomplicated (PY and LB)

This item is used to rate the toxic effects of alcohol during acute intoxication. Check for: disinhibition, argumentativeness, aggressiveness, impaired judgement and attention, lability; and irritability; slurred speech, unsteady gait, tremor, poor co-ordination, conjunctival injection, difficulty standing, flushed face, decreased level of consciousness, nystagmus, without the complications in **11.029 - 11.031**, only when intoxicated.

Such neurological toxic effects are typically dose related and vary with the direction of change in the subject's blood alcohol (i.e. increasing or decreasing).

11.029 Trauma, bodily injury due to alcohol (PY and LB)

11.030 Hematemesis, inhalation, other complications (PY and LB)

Medical complications such as hematemesis, inhalation of vomit should be rated here.

11.031 Change of consciousness due to alcohol (PY and LB)

Delirium or fits, as toxic rather than withdrawal effects, should be rated 3 at this item, not at item **11.028**.

11.032 Current drinking

This item indicates the current state of R's drinking.

11.033 Age at first onset of alcohol dependence

The item definition in the PSE10 text is comprehensive. The intention is to allow the establishment of the age of onset of a group of dependence symptoms according to the criteria stated. This age will often be an estimate, based on R's memory for the contiguity of symptoms some time previously. Always enter an age, even if approximate, if this is feasible.

11.034 Age at end of alcohol dependence

See item **11.033**. The same considerations apply.

11.035 Age at first onset of period of harm from alcohol

See item **11.033**. The same considerations apply.

11.036 Age at end of period of harm from alcohol

See item **11.033**. The same considerations apply.

List of withdrawal, toxic (neurological) effects and toxic dysfunctional behaviors due to alcohol.

Although the following symptoms have been referred to in the appropriate items, above, they are summarized here for convenience.

Withdrawal effects:

Tremor of the outstretched hands, tongue or eyelids.
Sweating.
Nausea, retching or vomiting.
Tachycardia or hypertension.
Psychomotor agitation.
Headache.
Insomnia.
Malaise or weakness.
Transient visual, tactile or auditory hallucinations or illusions.
Grand mal convulsions.

Toxic effects (neurological):

Unsteady gait.
Difficulty standing.
Slurred speech.
Nystagmus.
Decreased level of consciousness (e.g. stupor, coma).
Flushed face.
Conjunctival injection.

Dysfunctional behavior:

Disinhibition.
Argumentativeness.
Aggression.

Lability of mood.
Impaired attention.
Impaired judgement.
Interference with personal functioning.

12 Use of substances other than alcohol

GENERAL POINTS ABOUT SECTION 12

Section 12 covers disorders associated with the use of nine classes of psychoactive substance. Item **12.001** allows a cut-off from the whole section. Item **12.005** allows a skip to **12.022** if only prescription drugs are used. Then there is an opportunity to obtain a general account of the use of psychoactive drugs. This forms the basis for the subsequent examination. Interviewers should be acquainted with the possible effects of the different drug classes and with local colloquial names for them.

Items **12.006 - 12.014** establish the frequency of drug taking for each of the nine classes. The Glossary definition for each of these items contains an account of the characteristics of the relevant class of drug. Schematic lists of their different toxic and withdrawal characteristics are provided at the end of the Section.

Provision is made for rating each item from **12.015** onwards separately for each class. It is not feasible to include differential information within the text of each item. If there is any doubt reference should be made to Glossary items **12.006 - 12.014**.

12.001   Lifetime abstention from drugs

The section begins with a general probe, allowing a full cut-off if psychoactive drugs have never been used or only on one or two occasions in a lifetime. Always continue if there is any doubt.

12.002   Prescribed opioids (PY and LB)

12.003   Prescribed sedatives, hypnotics, anxiolytics (PY and LB)

12.004   Prescribed stimulants (PY and LB)

These three questions deal with prescription drugs that have potential for misuse. Enter the code that provides the best approximation of how often the subject has used prescribed opioids (**12.001**), prescribed sedative-hypnotics (**12.002**) and/or prescribed stimulants (**12.003**) under a doctor's prescription during the past year (PY) or previously (LB). If prescription drugs were used daily for less than one month, code 'monthly' or 'less than monthly.' If they were used for a longer period and discontinued, code frequency during heaviest period (e.g. daily).

12.005   Use of drugs on and outside prescription (PY and LB)

This item establishes whether drugs have been used according to prescription only (skip to **12.022**), or also outside prescription. If both legal (prescription) and illegal sources have been used, combine the quantities in subsequent estimates of frequency and quantity.

INTRODUCTORY PROBES

If illegal drugs have been used, or drugs have been taken outside of prescription, use introductory probes to obtain a general history and recent use of psychoactive substances. It is not necessary to repeat questions later if the answers have already been obtained.

First obtain a general account of the pattern of drug use and any effects or problems, both during the past year and before. Formulate the periods of heaviest and/or most problematic use. The probes should be used to help R give a spontaneous account. Usually only one or a few drugs will have been used. These are designated - [DRUG] or [DRUG/S] - in the text.

12.006 - 12.014   Frequency of drug use during period

Estimate the frequency of psychoactive substance use for both licit and illicit drugs. Prescription drugs are sometimes used in amounts exceeding a doctor's prescription, or are sought because of their psychoactive properties even though there is no medical reason to use them. Inquire about each drug class first, then make specific inquiry, using the terms for particular drugs, their effects and associated behaviors that are familiar in R's culture, community and social group.

12.006   Opioids (PY and LB)

Opioid is the generic term applied to alkaloids from the opium poppy and their synthetic analogues. The most commonly used opioids (such as morphine, heroin, codeine, hydromorphine, methadone, and meperidine) produce analgesia, mood changes (such as euphoria, which may change to apathy or dysphoria), respiratory depression, drowsiness, psychomotor retardation, slurred speech, impaired concentration or memory and impaired judgement. Over time, opioids induce tolerance and neuroadaptive changes that are responsible for rebound hyperexcitability when the drug is withdrawn.

Withdrawal symptoms include craving, malaise, anxiety, dysphoria, yawning, sweating, piloerection (waves of gooseflesh), dilated pupils, tachycardia, hypertension, lacrimation, rhinorrhoea, insomnia, nausea, vomiting, muscle aches and cramps, and fever.

With short-acting drugs such as morphine or heroin, withdrawal symptoms may appear within 8 to 12 hours after the last dose of the drug, reach a peak at 48 to 72 hours, and clear after 7 to 10 days. With longer-acting drugs, such as methadone, onset may not occur until 1 to 3 days after the last dose; symptoms peak between the third and eighth day and may persist for several weeks.

The numerous physical effects of opioid use (usually caused by intravenous injection) include: hepatitis B, hepatitis C, HIV infection, septicaemia, endocarditis, pneumonia and lung abscess, thrombophlebitis, and rhabdomyolosis. Psychological and social impairment is prominent.

12.007 Cannabinoids (PY and LB)

Cannabinoid is a generic term used to denote the various psychoactive preparations of the marijuana (hemp) plant, cannabis sativa. These include marijuana leaf (known as grass, weed or reefers), bhang, hashish (derived from the resin of the flowering heads of the plant) and hash oil. Cannabis is usually smoked. THC and its metabolites can be detected in the urine for several weeks after use.

Cannabis intoxication produces a feeling of euphoria, lightness of the limbs and talkativeness. It impairs driving and the performance of other complex, skilled activities; it produces decrements in immediate recall, attention span, reaction time, learning ability, motor coordination, depth perception, peripheral vision, time sense (the subject typically has a sensation of slowed time) and signal detection. Other signs of intoxication include excessive anxiety, suspiciousness or paranoid ideas in some and euphoria or apathy in others; impaired judgement, conjunctival injection, increased appetite, dry mouth, and tachycardia. Cannabis is sometimes consumed with alcohol, a combination that is additive in its effects.

There is some evidence that cannabis use can precipitate relapse in psychotic symptoms. Acute anxiety and panic states and acute delusional states, usually remitting within several days, have been reported with cannabis intoxication.

12.008 Sedatives, hypnotics and anxiolytics (PY and LB)

Sedatives, hypnotics and anxiolytics comprise a group of central nervous system depressants that have the capacity to relieve anxiety, and induce calmness and sleep. Several such drugs also induce amnesia and muscle relaxation, and some have anti-convulsant properties. Major classes of sedative/hypnotics include the benzodiazepines and the barbiturates. Also included are chloral hydrate, acetylcarbromal, glutethimide, methyprylon, ethchlorvynol, ethinamate, meprobamate, and methaqualone.

Barbiturates have a narrow therapeutic-to-toxic dosage range and are lethal in overdosage. Tolerance develops rapidly and the liability for physical dependence and abuse is high. Chloral hydrate, acetylcarbromal, glutethimide, methyprylon, ethchlorvynol, and ethinamate also have a high liability for physical dependence and abuse, and are highly lethal in overdosage.

All sedatives impair concentration, memory, and coordination. Other frequent effects are hangover, slurred speech, incoordination, unsteady gait, drowsiness, dry mouth, decreased gastrointestinal motility, and lability of mood. Sedatives occasionally produce a paradoxical reaction of excitement or rage. They shorten the time before onset of sleep but they suppress REM sleep. Withdrawal of the drug gives a rebound of REM sleep and deterioration of sleep patterns. In consequence, patients who are given a hypnotic over a long period can become psychologically and physically dependent on the drug even when they never exceed the prescribed dose. Withdrawal reactions can be severe, and they may occur after no more than several weeks of moderate use of sedative, hypnotic, or anxiolytic drugs.

Symptoms of withdrawal include anxiety, irritability, insomnia (often with nightmares), nausea or vomiting, tachycardia, sweating, orthostatic hypotension, hallucinatory misperceptions, muscle cramps, tremors and myoclonic twitches, hyper-reflexia, and grand mal seizures that may progress to fatal status epilepticus. A withdrawal delirium may develop, usually within one week after cessation or significant reduction in dosage.

Long-term sedative abuse is likely to produce impairments in memory, verbal and nonverbal learning, speed, and coordination that last long after detoxification and, in some, result in a permanent amnestic disorder.

12.009   Cocaine (PY and LB)

In SCAN, stimulant use disorders are subdivided into those due to the use of cocaine and those due to the use of other stimulants (item **12.010**). Cocaine shares the general properties of stimulants.

Cocaine is a powerful central nervous system stimulant used for euphoria or wakefulness. Repeated use produces dependence. Cocaine ("coke") is often sold as white, translucent, crystalline flakes or powder ("snuff", "snow"). The powder is sniffed ("snorting"), producing effects in one to three minutes; they last for about 30 minutes. Combined opioid and cocaine abusers are likely to inject cocaine intravenously. Cocaine may be ingested orally, often with alcohol. "Freebasing" refers to increasing the potency of cocaine by extracting pure cocaine alkaloid, the free base, and then inhaling the heated vapors through a cigarette or water pipe. The procedure is dangerous because the mixture is explosive and highly flammable.

"Crack" is alkaloidal cocaine (free base) that is sold as pure beige crystals already suitable for smoking. (Crack refers to the crackling sound the crystals make when they are heated). An intense "high" appears four to six seconds after crack is inhaled, but effects last only five to seven minutes. Mood then rapidly descends into dysphoria, and the user must repeat the process in order to regain the exhilaration and euphoria of the high. Overdosage appears to be more frequent with crack than with other forms of cocaine abuse.

Smoking cocaine produces a "rush" - an early feeling of elation or disappearance of anxiety, with exaggerated feelings of competence and self-esteem. It also interferes with judgement, so the user is likely to perform irresponsible, illegal, or dangerous activities without regard for consequences. Speech is pressured or even disjointed and incoherent. With large amounts, and especially if taken intravenously, the user experiences a "crash" - elation gives way to apprehension, ideas of reference, ringing in the ears, persecutory delusions, "snow lights" (hallucinations or pseudohallucinations resembling the twinkling of sunlight on frozen snow) or other hallucinations.

Acute toxic reactions may occur in both the naive experimenter and the chronic abuser of cocaine. They include a panic-like delirium, hyperpyrexia, hypertension (sometimes with subdural or subarachnoid hemorrhage), cardiac arrhythmias, myocardial infarct, cardiovascular collapse, seizures, status epilepticus, and death.

12.010   Stimulants (PY and LB)

A stimulant is any agent that activates, enhances or increases central nervous system renewal activity. These drugs include the amphetamines, cocaine, caffeine, and other xanthines, and synthetic diet suppressants such as methylphenidate. Other drugs have stimulant effects which are not their primary action but which may be manifest in high doses or other chronic use; they include antidepressives, anticholinergics and certain opioids. Cocaine is rated separately from other stimulants (see item **12.009**).

Symptoms suggestive of intoxication with stimulants include tachycardia, pupillary dilation, elevated blood pressure, hyper-reflexia, sweating, chills, nausea or vomiting, abnormal behavior such as fighting, grandiosity, hypervigilance, agitation and impaired judgement. A delirium developing within 24 hours of use occurs in some users. Chronic use commonly induces personality and behavior changes such as impulsivity, aggressivity, irritability, and suspiciousness. Amphetamine and related drugs induce psychotic reactions. These most commonly take the form of a delirium, developing within 24 hours of use, and delusional disorder, developing shortly after use of the drug during a period of long-term use of moderate or high doses. Rapidly developing persecutory delusions are characteristic.

Cessation of intake after prolonged or heavy use may produce a withdrawal reaction, with depressed mood, fatigue, sleep disturbance and increased dreaming.

12.011   Hallucinogens (PY and LB)

Hallucinogens are chemical agents which induce alterations in perception, thinking and feeling that resemble those of the functional psychoses without producing the gross impairment of memory and orientation characteristic of the organic syndromes. Examples include lysergic acid diethylamide (LSD), dimethyltryptamine (DMT), psilocin, mescaline, 3-4-methylenedioxyamphetamine (MDA), 3-4-methylenedioxy-methamphetamine (MDMA or Ecstasy). Phencyclidine (PCP) is recorded separately in SCAN (see item **12.012**).

Most hallucinogens are taken orally; DMT, however, is sniffed or smoked. Use is typically episodic; long-term, frequent use is extremely rare. Effects are noted within 20 to 30 minutes after ingestion: pupillary dilatation, blood pressure elevation, tachycardia, tremor, hyper-reflexia, and the psychedelic phase consisting of euphoria or mixed mood changes, visual illusions and altered perceptions, a blurring of boundaries between self and non-self, and sometimes a feeling of unity with the cosmos. After four or five hours, that phase is replaced with ideas of reference, increased awareness of the inner self, and a sense of magical control.

In addition to the hallucinosis that is regularly produced, adverse effects are frequent and include: (1) bad trips; (2) post-hallucinogen perception disorder or flashbacks; (3) delusional disorder, which generally follows a bad trip; the perceptual changes abate but the subject becomes convinced that his perceptual distortions correspond with reality; the delusional state may last only a day or two, or it may persist, and (4) affective or mood disorder, consisting of anxiety, depression, or mania occurring shortly after hallucinogen use and persisting for more than 24 hours; typically subjects feel that they can never be normal again and express concern that they have damaged their brain by taking the drug.

12.012 Phencyclidine (PY and LB)

Phencyclidine (PCP) is also hallucinogenic, but in addition, exerts both stimulant and depressant actions. Its use is recorded separately in SCAN.

PCP may be taken orally, intravenously, or by sniffing, but it is usually smoked. Effects begin within five minutes and peak at about 30 minutes. At first, the user feels euphoria, body warmth and tingling, floating sensations, and a feeling of calm isolation. Auditory and visual hallucinations may appear as well as altered body image, distorted perceptions of space and time, delusions and disorganization of thought. Accompanying neurological and physiological symptoms are dose related: hypertension, vertical or horizontal nystagmus, ataxia, dysarthria, elevated blood pressure, grimacing, saturation, hyper-reflexia, diminished responsiveness to pain, muscle rigidity, hyperacusis, and seizures.

Effects last for four to six hours although it may take one or two days for the user to feel completely back to his usual self. During the immediate recovery period there may be self-destructive or violent behavior. PCP delirium, PCP delusional disorder, and PCP mood disorder have been observed. As with the hallucinogens, it is not known whether such psychoses are specific drug effects or a manifestation of pre-existing vulnerability.

12.013 Volatile substances (PY and LB)

Volatile substances vaporize at ambient temperatures. Those inhaled for psychoactive use (also called inhalants) include glue, aerosol, paints, industrial solvents, lacquer thinners, gasoline, and cleaning fluids. Some substances are directly toxic to liver, kidney or heart, and some produce peripheral neuropathy or progressive brain degeneration.

The user typically soaks a rag with inhalant and places it over mouth and nose, or puts the inhalant in a paper bag which is then put over the face (inducing anoxia as well as intoxication). Signs of intoxication include belligerence, assaultiveness, lethargy, psychomotor impairment, euphoria, impaired judgement, dizziness, nystagmus, blurred vision or diplopia, slurred speech, tremors, unsteady gait, hyper-reflexia, muscle weakness, stupor, or coma.

12.014 Other and unknown (PY and LB)

Use the "other" category to inquire about substances that may be unique to a particular culture, community or social group.

If it is impossible to ascertain the drug or drugs used, rate the effects under this item.

12.015.1-9 Most recent use

This item is rated for each substance used during the present year. This information, when considered in relation to urine drug screens, may be useful in estimating the veracity of self-report information provided by the subject.

RATING CLASSES OF DRUGS

Each class of drug is given a number from 1-9. The following items refer to problems that may or may not be relevant to all classes. It is important to ask them all in order to establish the pattern of effects for each drug taken, irrespective of what is expected. However, it is only necessary to make inquiries about those classes that have already been established as used by R. The other boxes should be left blank.

12.016 - 12.021 Method of administration of drug during past year (PY and LB)

These items all have the same rating scheme: 0. not used; 1. used, but not the usual method; 2. the usual method of administration during the year. Frequency has already been rated and need not be taken into account here. If for example, cocaine has been used only once during the year, and on this occasion was injected intravenously, the rating on **12.016.4** is 2.

12.022.1-9 Subjective need for drug

This aspect of drug dependence is manifested by a persistent preoccupation and subjective need for a psychoactive substance. R feels uneasy at times or in places where the drug is not available. Often this symptom is identified as drug craving. Rate 0 if there is no expressed need, or if the substance is needed only for medicinal reasons. Rate 1 if R experiences mild to moderate craving or uneasiness when the drug is not available. Rate 2 if perceived need is intrusive.

Be particularly careful about asking questions **12.022 - 12.029**, if use of drugs has been low and non-problematic. There is no need to ask again if the questions have already been answered in the general enquiry.

12.023.1-9 Impaired capacity to abstain or cut drug use (PY and LB)

R expresses a desire to stop drug use, but reports that repeated attempts have been unsuccessful. Typically these attempts include rules and other stratagems to avoid drugs entirely or to limit the frequency of drug use. One way to judge the degree of impaired control is to determine whether R has made repeated attempts to limit the quantity of drug consumption, using such tactics as making rules or imposing limits on access to drugs. The more these attempts have failed, the more the subject manifests inability to abstain. Resumption of drug use after seeking professional help for a drug problem, or joining a mutual help group such as Narcotics Anonymous, is evidence of lack of success. Rate 2 if R failed to abstain or cut down for a month or more. Rate 1 if R was able to abstain or cut down for a month or more, but only with the help of treatment, self-help groups, or controlled environment.

12.024.1-9   Impaired capacity to control drug once use started (PY and LB)

Diminished ability consistently to choose whether or not to use a psychoactive substance, or consistently to choose when to stop after having begun to use the substance, is a cardinal sign of dependence. R is aware of an impaired capacity to control drug use in terms of the amounts consumed and termination of use. This impaired control includes the failure to control spontaneous onset of substance use and inability to stop before intoxication levels are attained. This behavior should be distinguished from situations in which the respondent's control over the onset or amount of drug use is strongly determined by social or cultural factors.

> **NOTE: The following items (11.025, 11.026, 11.034 and 11.038) refer to harm caused by drugs. For harm to be rated the nature of harm should be clearly identifiable and must occur for month at a stretch or repeatedly over a year.**

12.025.1-9   Social problems due to drug taking (PY and LB)

Drug use is associated with a wide variety of social problems that result from the direct effects of intoxication (e.g. absence from work or inability to drive an automobile), the indirect effects from intoxication (e.g. criticism by employer or spouse) or the cumulative effects of chronic substance abuse (e.g. legal problems or marital discord). The social consequences of drug use are sometimes affected by the respondent's age, gender and culture. In some cases (e.g. a first time marijuana user receiving a long prison sentence), these mitigating factors should be taken into account in rating the severity of problems due to drugs. In general, drug intoxication meets with more serious social sanctions when the user is younger and female, and when substance use takes place in a society that imposes severe legal and social sanctions on the possession and use of psychoactive drugs. The seriousness of a social problem should be judged according to age, gender or culture-specific norms. Social problems should be rated only when they are the result of impaired judgement or dysfunctional behavior that are a direct consequence of drug use.

12.026.1-9   Legal problems due to drug taking (PY and LB)

Drug taking can be the cause of legal problems of varying severity, either directly related to drug taking (e.g. getting arrested for drug trafficking, being prosecuted because of possession or use of drugs, being arrested for theft to obtain drugs, being put in jail for prostitution to obtain drugs, getting arrested for the production of drugs for personal use, being convicted of break and entry of a pharmacy to obtain drugs) or indirectly (e.g. being imprisoned because of an inability to pay debts due to drug payments, being divorced due to drug taking, being sued for an inability to fulfill major financial or role obligations such as child support because of drug taking). Legal problems should be rated only when they are the result of impaired judgement or dysfunctional behavior that are a direct consequence of drug use.

12.027.1-9 Persistent drug taking after social/legal harm

The key aspect of this symptom is the persistence of drug use in spite of knowledge of social harm, such as legal problems or complaints by spouse. This indicates that drug use is given a higher priority than other activities, in spite of its negative consequences. If the subject stopped using drugs, cut down on the frequency or amount of use, or otherwise made successful efforts to avoid future problems, then score this question as 0 (No). If these changes were only temporary, after which the subject returned to the same pattern of drug use, score 1 (Yes). If R does not realize or is not aware of harm, rate 0.

12.028.1-9 Failure to fulfill major role obligations (PY and LB)

A common symptom of dependence is the inability to fulfill major role obligations because of drug use or intoxication. If there is evidence that drug use is only incidental to lack of role performance, code this item zero.

12.029.1-9 Risk-taking behavior with drugs (PY and LB)

Use examples that are appropriate to R's age, gender and culture. Severity of risk is rated according to the nature of the risk, whether it involves self or others.

The rating should be made on assessment of risk, not simply of quantity of drug taken. For example, does R know the limits within which he or she can use a particular drug or drugs, and act within them? Rate (1) if there has been risk-taking behavior during the period. Rate (2) if harm has actually occurred to self or others because of drugtaking.

CUT-OFF POINT

12.030.1-9 Salience of drug-related activities (PY and LB)

Substance use is given a higher priority than other activities, in spite of its negative consequences. R shows diminished responsiveness to the normal processes of informal social control. Substance use or drug intoxication interferes with R's ability to conform to tacit social rules governing activities, such as keeping appointments or caring for children, that are typically expected by the user's reference group.

12.031.1-9 Time involved in drug-related activities (PY and LB)

The amount of time or effort devoted to obtaining, using or recovering from substance use is rated. If R spends a great deal of time in drug-related activities, such as a month or more of daily or continuous involvement, rate (2). If less time is spent in drug use, rate (1).

12.032.1-9   Narrowing of drug-taking pattern (PY and LB)

Narrowing is the tendency of substance use to become progressively stereotyped around a prescribed routine of customs and rituals. It is characterized by increasing facility in performing the ritual, habitual use of a regime of doses, and lack of variation in time, place or manner of substance use. Rate 0 if drug use is not associated with habitual customs or rituals. Rate 1 if there is some regularity to the drug use pattern. Rate 2 if the pattern is fixed with regard to time, place or manner of use.

12.033.1-9   Tolerance to drugs (PY and LB)

Tolerance involves a gradual decrease in response to a particular dose of drug. Increased doses are required to achieve effects originally produced by lower doses, or a constant dosage is found to produce reduced effects. Tolerance may be physical, behavioral or psychological. A clear example would be the consumption without significant impairment of amounts of cocaine, heroin or barbiturates that might have gravely impaired function or even proved lethal at an earlier date.

Reversed tolerance is rated 3. This is the development of sensitivity to doses of drug that formerly would have been tolerated without toxic effects. It can occur after cutting down on drugtaking or while continuing at a steady level.

12.034.1-9   Psychological and mental health problems due to drugtaking (PY and LB)

Drug use is associated with a wide variety of psychological and mental health problems that result from the direct effects of intoxication (e.g. aggressive behavior), the sequelae of intoxication (e.g. depression, delusional symptoms) or the cumulative effects of drug abuse (e.g. insomnia, depression, paranoid thinking).

The attribution of cause is made in this item. If more than one type of symptom is caused (for example, hallucinations and depression) choose the most severe. The scale is in order of severity of type of symptom, with 9 (memory problems) the most severe. The severity of the mental symptoms themselves is not rated here but in the relevant Sections of PSE10. Onset of psychotic symptoms must have been within 2 weeks of the last occasion of substance use and last for more than 48 hours but less than 6 months.

Memory and other cognitive problems, and any attribution to drugs as their cause, are rated in Section 21. See items **21.113, 21.117, 21.121, 21.122**. Delirium, with or without fits, is rated 3 at item **12.040** and, in more detail, in Section 20.

Delirium and fits as withdrawal symptoms are rated 3 at item **12.040** and, as toxic symptoms at item **12.043**. All cognitive problems should be rated, in more detail, in Section 21 (see items **21.113, 21.117, 21.121, 21.122**).

12.035.1-9 Onset of drug-induced mental health problems

The purpose of this item is to differentiate where possible between psychiatric problems that are associated with intoxication, drug withdrawal, or neither. This is done by indicating the circumstances under which symptoms directly attributed to drugs had their onset.

12.036.1-9 Interference due to drug-induced symptoms (PY and LB)

Rate the degree of interference resulting from the worst mental health symptoms coded in item **12.034.1-9**. Exclude social problems and physical health problems rated at items **12.025** and **12.038** as well as neglect of obligations and time lost due to drug use rated in **12.028** and **12.031**. Exclude physiological effects of intoxication and withdrawal.

12.037.1-9 Persistent drug-taking after mental harm (PY and LB)

The key aspect of this dependence symptom is the persistence of drug taking in spite of knowledge of any mental harm caused by it, such as depressive symptoms or hallucinations. If the subject stopped drug taking, cut down on the frequency or amount of drug use, or otherwise made successful efforts to avoid future problems, then score this question 0 (No). If these changes were only temporary, after which the subject returned to the same drug use pattern, score 1 (Yes). If R does not realize or is not aware of harm, rate 0.

12.038.1-9 Physical health problems and functional disability due to drug-taking (PY and LB)

Substance use is associated with a wide variety of physical health problems (see notes at end of Section). Some are direct toxic effects due to the pharmacological properties of the substance and the dose taken. Toxic effects are rated below at **12.043.1-9**. Other problems are secondary to drug use, for example accidents, trauma, infections and, perforated nasal septum. Still others result from chronic intoxication on different body systems. Rate severity of health problems according to the degree of functional disability: 1 refers to mild physical illness or functional disability; 2 refers to physical illness of moderate severity. Rate 3 if R's drug-related problems are life threatening.

12.039.1-9 Persistent drug-taking after physical harm (PY and LB)

The key aspect of this dependence symptom is the persistence of drug use in spite of knowledge of physical harm, such as hepatitis, overdose or traumatic injury. This indicates that drug use is given a higher priority than being healthy. If R stopped using drugs, cut down on the frequency of drug use, or otherwise made successful efforts to avoid future problems, score this question 0 (No). If no reduction was made, or changes were only temporary, after which the subject returned to the same pattern of substance use, score 1 (Yes). If R does not realize or is not aware of harm, rate 0.

12.040.1-9 Drug withdrawal problems (PY and LB)

Withdrawal symptoms do not necessarily occur together, they vary in degree of severity, and are often specific for a given substance. The physical effects tend to occur after repeated, and usually prolonged and/or high-dose use of many but not all psychoactive substances. Withdrawal symptoms should not be coded if they can be accounted for by a medical disorder unrelated to substance use, of by another mental disorder. It is essential, therefore, to ask specific questions related to the action of the drug used. See items **12.006 - 12.014** and notes at the end of the Section for details of withdrawal effects for each type of drug. In addition to physical withdrawal symptoms, psychological disturbances (e.g. anxiety, depression) and sleep disturbance are also common features. While it may be sufficient to gauge the manifestation of mild withdrawal symptoms on the basis of brief periods of abstinence (e.g. after a typical night of sleep), some chronic drug users have never had a long enough period of abstinence to permit withdrawal to occur. It is therefore important to ask if the subject ever had a period of abstinence longer than several days.

12.041.1-9 Multiple drug withdrawal state

12.042.1-9 Drug-taking to relieve or to avoid withdrawal symptoms (PY and LB)

R uses drugs with the intention of relieving or avoiding the onset of withdrawal symptoms (**12.040.1-9**) and with an awareness that this strategy is effective; for example, a morning injection of heroin specifically in order to relieve nausea, or to avoid its anticipated onset.

NB: **For rating acute toxic effects of drugs ensure that the symptoms or signs are not better accounted for by another medical disorder unrelated to the substance use or by another mental or behavioral disorder.**

12.043.1-9 Toxic effects of drugs (PY and LB)

Rate here the severity of dysfunctional behaviors and of toxic effects of drugs, either during the year or at examination. See the notes at the end of the Section and the definitions of toxicity and dysfunctional behaviors given for items **12.006 - 12.014**. A rating of (1) is reserved for mild to moderate severity, whether psychological, physical or behavioral. Effects that severely interfere with everyday activities, are rated (2), but must include at least one item each from behavioral and physical (neurological) checklist. A rating of (3) is used only to indicate the presence of delirium or coma.

12.044.1-9 Current drugtaking

This item indicates the current state (e.g. the past month) of R's drugtaking.

12.045.1-9   Age at first onset of drug dependence

The item definition in the PSE10 text is comprehensive. The intention is to allow the establishment of the age of onset of a group of dependence symptoms according to the criteria stated. This age will often be an estimate, based on R's memory for the contiguity of symptoms some time previously. Always enter an age, even if approximate, if this is feasible.

12.046.1-9   Age, end of drug dependence

See item **12.045**. The same considerations apply.

12.047.1-9   Age at first onset of period of harm from drug taking

See item **12.045**. The same considerations apply.

12.048.1-9   Age, end of period of harm from drug taking

See item **12.045**. The same considerations apply.

12.049 - 12.058   Optional checklist

This is used to rate the effects of using drugs, whether or not on prescription, that are not dealt with elsewhere in Section 12.

12.059 - 12.104   Optional appendix (tobacco)

The items in this appendix mirror those in Sections 11 and 12, modified for the effects of tobacco.

CHECKLIST OF WITHDRAWAL AND TOXIC EFFECTS BY CLASS OF DRUG

[The number identifying each class is the code used to rate its withdrawal effects in item **12.040.1-9** and its toxic effects in item **12.043.1-9**]

1.   Opioids

Withdrawal

Craving
Dilated pupils
Tachycardia, hypertension
Anxiety, agitation, sleep problems
Salivation, lacrimation, sweating, rhinorrhoea or sneezing
Goose flesh (piloerection), or recurrent chills
Muscle ache and cramps, abdominal cramps
Fever, malaise

Dysphoria
Nausea and vomiting
Diarrhoea
Yawning
Restless sleep

Toxicity

Death
Stupor, lethargy, drowsiness, coma
Respiratory depression
Disinhibition
Impaired judgement
Slurred speech
Infectious hepatitis, subacute bacterial endocarditis septicaemia, abscesses in organs
Apathy, hypophoria, dysphoria
Pupillary constriction (except in anoxia from severe overdose when pupillary dilation occurs)
Impaired concentration and memory
Slowed speech and motor activity
Bradycardia, hypotension, hypothermia
Loss of interest in and performance of sex

Dysfunctional behavior

Apathy and sedation
Disinhibition
Psychomotor retardation
Impaired attention
Impaired judgement
Interference with personal functioning

2. **Cannabinoids**

Withdrawal

Possible symptoms in cessation after prolonged high dose usage, but no criteria can be laid down.

Toxicity

Excessive anxiety
Suspiciousness or paranoid ideas
Impaired sense of time and short-term memory
Increased reaction time

Dysfunctional behavior or perceptual disturbances

Euphoria and disinhibition
Anxiety or agitation
Suspiciousness or paranoid ideation
Temporal slowing (a sense that time is passing very slowly, and/or the person is experiencing a rapid flow of ideas)
Impaired judgement
Impaired attention
Impaired reaction time
Auditory, visual or tactile illusions
Hallucinations with preserved orientation
Depersonalization
Derealization
Interference with personal functioning
Depersonalization
Derealization
Tachycardia
Conjunctival injection
Increased appetite, weight gain
Dry mouth
Impaired judgement
Euphoria and disinhibition
Impaired attention
Impaired driving and other complex tasks, including learning
Depression
Precipitated relapse in schizophrenia
Auditory, visual or tactile illusions
Reduced motivation, increased apathy
Hallucination with perceived orientation

3. Sedatives, hypnotics, anxiolytics

Withdrawal

Nausea, vomiting
Weakness, malaise
Sweating
Tachycardia, high blood pressure
Postural hypotension
Headache
Insomnia
Tremor of outstretched hands, tongue or eyelids
Transient visual, tactile or auditory hallucinations or illusions
Paranoid ideation
Psychomotor agitation

Fits (grand mal), delirium

Toxicity

CNS depression, stupor, coma, death (overdose) from respiratory depression
Clouded consciousness
Poor coordination, unsteady gait, difficulty standing
Impaired psychomotor performance
Slurred speech
Nystagmus
Erythematous skin lesion or blisters

Dysfunctional behavior

Apathy
Abusiveness
Lability of mood, garrulousness, ,
Euphoria and behavioral disinhibition
Hostility and aggression,
Anterograde amnesia, , confusion
Impaired concentration and memory
Interference with personal functioning

4. **Cocaine**

Withdrawal

Craving for cocaine
Anxiety, restlessness
Irritability, anger
Difficulty concentrating
Increased appetite, food consumption and weight gain
Slowed heart rate
Headaches
Drowsiness, malaise
Lethargy and fatigue
psychomotor retardation, agitation
Depression, dysphoria
Inability to experience pleasure (hypophoria)
Poor sleep, exhaustion
Bizarre or unpleasant dreams

Toxicity

Psychomotor agitation

Tremors, delirium, coma, convulsions, death
Tachycardia, cardiac arrhythmia, chest pain, coronary artery spasm, infarction, cardiomyopathy
Exhaustion
Precipitation of mania
Impaired judgement
Hyperpyrexia
Hypertension, stroke (sometimes hypotension)
Sweating and chills
Malnutrition,
Nausea or vomiting
Muscular weakness
Evidence of weight loss
Pupillary dilatation
Deterioration in general hygiene and social and financial functioning

Dysfunctional behavior or perceptual abnormalities

Euphoria and sensation of increased energy
Panic
Hypervigilance
Grandiose beliefs or actions
Abusiveness or aggression
Argumentativeness
Irresponsible actions
Lability of mood
Repetitive stereotyped behaviors
Auditory, visual or tactile illusions
Hallucinations usually with intact orientation
Paranoid ideation
Interference with personal functioning
Hostility, aggression, violence
Paranoia, hallucinations, delusions of persecution

5. **Stimulants other than cocaine**

Withdrawal

Lethargy and fatigue
Psychomotor retardation or agitation
Craving for stimulant drugs
Increased appetite
Insomnia or hypersomnia
Bizarre or unpleasant dreams

Toxic (neurological) effects

Tachycardia (sometimes bradycardia)
Cardiac arrhythmias
Hypertension (sometimes hypotension)
Sweating and chills
Nausea or vomiting
Evidence of weight loss
Pupillary dilatation
Psychomotor agitation (sometimes retardation)
Muscular weakness
Chest pain
Convulsions

Dysfunctional behavior or perceptual abnormalities

Euphoria and sensation of increased energy
Hypervigilance
Grandiose beliefs or actions
Abusiveness or aggression
Argumentativeness
Lability of mood
Repetitive stereotyped behaviors
Auditory, visual or tactile illusions
Hallucinations usually with intact orientation
Paranoid ideation
Interference with personal functioning

6. **Hallucinogens and**

7. **PCP**

Withdrawal

None

Toxicity

Raised blood pressure, tachycardia
Palpitations
Sweating and chills
Blurred vision
Pupillary dilatation
Incoordination
Tremor, increased reflexes

Dysfunctional behaviors or perceptual abnormalities

Anxiety and fearfulness, depression,
Suspiciousness
Altered perceptions, modes of thinking and feeling
Auditory, visual or tactile illusions or hallucinations occurring in a state of full wakefulness and alertness
Negative autoscopy
Delusions ('bad trips')
Flashbacks
Depersonalization
Derealization
Paranoid ideation
Ideas of reference
Lability of mood, elation
Hyperactivity
Impulsive acts
Impaired attention
Interference with personal functioning

8. Nicotine

Withdrawal

Craving for tobacco (or other nicotine-containing products)
Malaise or weakness
Anxiety
Dysphoric mood
Irritability or restlessness
Insomnia
Increased appetite
Increased cough
Mouth ulceration
Difficulty concentrating

Toxicity

Nausea or vomiting
Sweating
Tachycardia
Cardiac arrhythmias

Dysfunctional behaviors or perceptual abnormalities

Lability of mood
Insomnia
Bizarre dreams
Derealization

Interference with personal functioning

9. **Volatile Substances**

Withdrawal

No criteria described or listed in ICD-10 DCR

Toxicity

Unsteady gait
Difficulty standing
Slurred speech
Nystagmus
Decreased level of consciousness (e.g. stupor, coma)
Muscle weakness
Blurred vision or diplopia

Dysfunctional behaviors or perceptual abnormalities

Aggression, abusiveness, argumentativeness
Apathy, lethargy,
Lability of mood
Impaired judgement
Impaired judgement
Impaired attention and memory
Psychomotor retardation
Interference with personal functioning

ROUTES OF ADMINISTRATION

Subcutaneous	Intravenous	Intramuscular
Opioids	Opioids	Opioids
Sedatives	Sedatives	
Cocaine	Cocaine	
Stimulants	Stimulants	
Hallucinogens (DMT)	Hallucinogens	
PCP	PCP	

Smoking

Opioids
Cocaine
Cannabinoids
PCP

Snorting or sniffing

Opioids
Cocaine
Volatiles
PCP

By mouth

Opioids
Cannabinoids
Sedatives
Cocaine (not very effective)
Stimulants
Hallucinogens
PCP

13   Factors influencing the manifestation of Part One symptoms

GENERAL POINTS ABOUT SECTION 13

The various subsections of Section 13 provide contextual material for Part One of SCAN and an opportunity to rate organic and other attributions of cause separately from earlier ratings of symptom presence and severity. A list of factors that may influence all of the symptoms rated throughout Part One can also be rated. The Section ends with an optional check list of stress and adjustment symptoms in which specific items that may have been influenced by adverse life events or traumas can be recorded.

13.001 - 13.016   Greatest cause of interference due to Part One symptoms

The interviewer is reminded to review earlier ratings of interference within each section of Part One. If several ratings are of an equal severity level, this is an opportunity to decide if one interference rating should be greater than other such ratings in order to indicate which group of symptoms was responsible for the greatest level of interference. If necessary re-rate interference items in Sections 2-12, e.g. **5.015, 6.027** etc.

13.017 - 13.031   Relationship of Part One symptoms and syndromes to each other

This is an opportunity for the examiner to make his/her own clinical judgement of which group of symptoms or syndrome is the most clinically significant throughout the period rated. Take account of all available information (time of onset, severity, degree of interference caused, the respondent's own opinion) as well as clinical judgement.

13.032   Positive activities/enjoyment irrespective of problems

Refer to text for the ratings.

FACTORS INFLUENCING THE MANIFESTATION OF SYMPTOMS IN SPECIFIED SECTIONS OF PART ONE DURING THE PERIOD

Both ICD-10 and DSM require the exclusion of attributions of "cause", particularly in relation to the judged effects of psychoactive substances and alcohol, other treatments, physical (or "organic") disease, and psychosocial stressors and adversity. Users of SCAN who wish to make use of such classification systems must therefore attempt to consider the grounds for making judgements of this kind. Although opportunities to do so at the item level are present for many items using the optional etiology scale and the etiology boxes, Section 13 allows the user to re-rate these at a syndromal level. The following criteria for rating attribution of cause should be used here and also for making item level attributions of etiology using the etiology scale and optional boxes.

NOTE: Users should establish that ratings of attribution can be made reliably. As far as is practicable, such attributional ratings should be delayed until the "causal" status of any attribution can be established with reasonable certainty:

Criteria for rating Attributions of Cause

(Taken from ICD-10, DCR).

If the following three criteria are met, a provisional attribution (i.e. rate 1) can be made:

There is objective evidence (from physical and neurological examination and laboratory tests) and/or history of cerebral disease, damage, or dysfunction, or of systematic physical disorder known to cause cerebral dysfunction, including hormonal disturbances (other than alcohol- or other psychoactive substance-related) and non-psychoactive drug effects.

There is a presumed relationship between the development (or marked exacerbation) of the underlying disease, damage, or dysfunction, and the mental disorder, the symptoms of which may have immediate onset or may be delayed.

There is insufficient evidence for an alternative causation of the mental disorder, e.g. strong family history of a clinically similar or related disorder.

Rate 1, if the above three criteria are satisfied. If not rate 0. If, in addition the following criterion can be met, the attribution can be regarded as more certain and rate 2. If in doubt, rate 8. Keep careful records of the evidence upon which ratings are based:

There is recovery from or significant improvement in the mental disorder following removal or improvement of the underlying presumed cause.

13.033 - 13.048   Rate certainty of attributions and quality of evidence available

Follow instructions in the SCAN Manual using the above criteria.

13.049 - 13.054   Rate nature of attribution

Record the item number corresponding to the Section rated (**13.017 - 13.031**). Record the nature of the attribution using the ICD-10 Chapter identifier and up to 3 digits. See Glossary Appendix for a list of well recognized causes. Leave blank if none. If the symptoms in the same Section of Part One have also caused interference with functioning, rate the effect of the attributed cause on the interference. For example, if the attribution has caused little interference with functioning rate 1, but if it has been directly responsible for severe to incapacitating interference rate 3. Up to three separate attributions can be rated. If two PERIODS were rated in Part One, these ratings apply to the left hand box (present state/episode). If more detailed rating is needed use the etiology scale and the optional etiology boxes.

13.055 - 13.128   Optional checklists: Stress and adjustment disorders - ICD-10 and DSM

The presence/severity of most of the listed items/symptoms may have been rated already in Sections 3, 4, 6, 7, 8, apart from a limited number of additional symptoms specific to stress reactions. In this part of the examination, the interviewer rates attributions of psychosocial influence and their supposed cause or causes in the form of threatening life events or traumas. Similar strict criteria to those employed in the rating of organic attributions should also be applied. In general, these attributions are only required for symptoms that are moderate or severe clinically (i.e. 2 or 3 on Scale I). Symptoms must have begun after R became aware of or experienced the stress or trauma. Certain symptoms can occur within a few minutes or hours; other symptoms may take days or weeks to develop. The reliability of these attributional ratings is uncertain and ideally informants should be sought both to confirm information about external factors and to report on those that R either denies or appears unable to recall. For some forms of stress disorder, duration need only be for a few hours and therefore the corresponding item/s will have been rated absent in earlier Sections of Part One. Begin by recording the putative cause of these symptoms.

13.129   Adequacy of ratings in Sections 2-12

This item should be carefully rated, taking into account two kinds of problem listed below. (These apply also to items **20.092, 24.031, 26.059**). The effect of such problems can be to limit the examiner's ability to explore the phenomena appropriately through the process of clinical cross-examination and thus limit the accuracy of the ratings made.

The number of items rated 8 is provided as a separate score for each Item Group in the output from SCAN. This overall adequacy rating will also be an important factor in assessing the value of the output.

Sources of information

- Language problems rated in Section 15.
- Abnormalities of speech rated in Section 24.
- Poor co-operation during the interview.
- Evasiveness, rated at **24.028.**
- Poor quality of information from case records or informants.

Rater's own problems

- Inadequate knowledge of language or (R's and that of records and informants).
- Lack of familiarity with R's culture, social class, etc.
- Lack of clinical experience.
- Lack of training in SCAN techniques.

13.130 - 13.138 Additional specified factors influencing the overall manifestation of symptoms throughout Part Two

Rate the judged effect of each of the possible influences listed. These ratings refer to attributions of cause that effect all of the symptoms rated in Part One. This may be useful where there are relatively few positively rated items throughout Part One and where the more detailed ratings of attributions (**13.017 - 13.031** and **13.033 - 13.048**) are not appropriate. If adverse life events or other traumatic circumstances have been rated, the detailed stress and adjustment disorder check lists should also be completed (**13.055 - 13.128**).

14 Screen for items in Part Two

GENERAL POINTS ABOUT SECTION 14

Part Two is optional, in the sense that many studies are carried out in populations where the frequency of psychotic and cognitive disorders is very low and do not form part of the objectives of the project. Selected survey interviewers, after special training, can use the shorter form of Part One. In all such studies, the selection of key items in the Screen can be used to record Part Two symptoms which might suggest a need for further investigation. Alternatively, the Screen can be used by a fully qualified interviewer to check whether it is necessary to proceed further.

If Part Two is used as well as the Screen, and some items are thus rated twice, the Part Two item will overwrite that in the Screen and be used by the CATEGO program.

15 Language deficits at examination

GENERAL POINTS ABOUT SECTION 15

Much of PSE10 is concerned with eliciting accurate descriptions of the respondent's mental state, in order to match them against the item concepts defined in this Glossary. The interviewer's skill in eliciting accurate descriptions will depend substantially on knowledge of R's language and dialect, familiarity with R's culture and social class and clinical experience and training in SCAN. Since much of the information on which ratings are based is subjective, and depends on an accurate description of mental experiences that may be strange, complex and difficult to put into words, the value of ratings depends on the respondent's ability (with help from a skilled interviewer) for clear verbal expression. This is particularly true of psychotic symptoms.

Section 15 allows a rating to be made of language problems that have been encountered during Part I of the interview. More than one of the eight items may be rated if present together. A rating of (1) provides a warning that subsequent ratings must be interpreted with caution. If any item in later sections is too difficult to rate because of language disorder, it is rated (5).

Any item rated (2) indicates that the interview is very unlikely to yield useful information about subjective symptoms. However, behavior, affect and speech (in more detail) can be rated, i.e. items **22.065** onwards.

If a combination of problems, each rateable as (1), adds up to an overall rating of 2, rate one of them (the most prominent) at (2) nevertheless, and skip to item **21.065**.

If there is any evidence for disorders in the autistic spectrum, which includes Asperger's syndrome and 'atypical' autism, always rate the cognitive and behavioral Sections 21 - 25, and the developmental disorders at items **27.012 - 27.019** of the Clinical History Schedule.

GENERAL POINTS ABOUT SECTIONS 16 - 19

These Sections are concerned with abnormal experiences and beliefs. They are arranged, both as to order and to content, for convenience of interviewing, not clarity of underlying theoretical ideas. Thus Sections 16 and 17 contain items that deal with delusional interpretations of the experiences. Sections 18 and 19 both contain items about 'primary' and 'secondary' phenomena. The first pages of each of the Sections 16 - 19 contain definitions that are relevant to all the others. The discussion of concepts of delusion, at the beginning of Section 19, is particularly relevant.

GENERAL POINTS ABOUT RATING

The main rating scale in Sections 16 - 19 is Scale II. The rating points are specified in the SCAN text, at the beginning of Section 16, and elaborated on the next page of the Glossary.

However, many items in these Sections have their own individual rating scales, which are specified within their item blocks. It should be noted that all symptom items can be rated at points 0, 8 and 9, using the definitions given in Scale I (and repeated in Scale II), whether or not these points are specified in the text.

Section 20 and 21 have their own rating techniques and Sections 22 - 24 use Rating Scale III.

RATING SEVERITY

The severity of a symptom can be assessed in terms of duration, persistence, degree of interference with mental functions, distress, impairment of everyday activities, effect on other people, and contact with services of various kinds. In SCAN, the approach is to measure clinical severity as far as possible. This is gauged by the duration and frequency of the symptom and the degree of interference with mental functions (intensity). Social and occupational performance, other people's reactions, and help - seeking behavior (all of which can be influenced by many other factors), can be assessed independently and an attribution as to whether they are caused by the symptom openly specified.

This discussion of the concept of 'severity' is quoted from the text concerned with ratings in Part One of SCAN but it applies also to Sections 16 - 19. In contradistinction to 'neurotic' and 'depressive' symptoms, however, 'psychotic' symptoms are relatively rare in the general population. A further point of difference is that, although they can be measured along a dimension of severity, it is less extensive than, for example, a symptom such as worrying or depressed mood. Psychotic symptoms may have severe implications or severe effects on mental functions, even when present relatively infrequently, and even when they appear to be mild.

The solution adopted in Rating Scale II is to measure clinical intensity according to either frequency (e.g. hallucinations) or duration (e.g. delusions). No attempt is made to define mild, moderate and severe versions of each symptom. This means that any rating of (1 - 3) is recognized by CATEGO5 as meeting the threshold for purposes of classification.

RATING SCALE II

0   This is a positive rating of absence. It does not mean 'not known' or 'uncertain whether present or not'. It can only be used if sufficient information is available to establish its accuracy.
1   Symptom definitely occurred during the period but was probably uncommon or transitory.
2   Symptom was definitely present, on multiple occasions or for part of the time, during the period.
3   Symptom was present more or less continuously throughout the period.
5   Language difficulty, rated as present in Section 15, makes replies difficult to interpret.
8   If, after an adequate examination, the interviewer is still not sure whether a symptom is present (rated 1 - 3) or absent (rated 0), the rating is (8). This is the only circumstance in which (8) is used. It should not be used to indicate a mild form of the symptom, or an inadequate examination.
9   This rating is only used if the information needed to rate an item is incomplete in some respect, for example because of language or cognitive disorder, or lack of cooperation, or because the interviewer forgot or was unable to probe sufficiently deeply. It is distinguished from (8) because the examination could not be (or was not) carried out adequately.

NB: In the case of delusions, the rating is made on the approximate length of time R was deluded during the PERIOD and on the continuity of the beliefs. A rating of (2) applies only if R is not continuously deluded.

ATTRIBUTIONAL SCALE (OPTIONAL)

For research purposes attributional ratings of Part Two items might be useful. For this purpose the attributional etiology scale may be used, keeping in mind the criteria for attribution as specified in Section 13. See Manual Section 1 for scale.

16 Perceptual disorders other than hallucinations

GENERAL POINTS ABOUT SECTION 16

The following general points should be read in conjunction with those for Sections 17, 18 and 19.

Many of the items in this section are concerned with symptoms that can occur in a delusional or non - delusional form. The distinction is made on the extent to which the respondent is aware of the abnormal nature of the perception or experience, particularly when seen through the eyes of others, and of its 'as if' quality which is unlike the experience, for example, of hallucinations. The delusions (items **16.012** and **16.013**) are 'secondary' or 'delusion - like' (see beginning of Section 19).

Sections 16 and 17 should always be rated independently of each other. Both kinds of experience can be present at the same time.

The course of the interview so far is likely to have indicated whether perceptual disorders are present.

Rating scale II should be used for all items.

16.001 Unusual perceptions

Probe for Section 16 symptoms. Skip from the Section if no evidence following adequate probing.

16.002 Changing perceptions

Include here any change in perception that is not included under items **16.003** and **16.004** (dulled and heightened perception). The subject may complain that objects change in shape or size or color or that people change their appearance. Once the symptom has disappeared it may be difficult for the subject to remember or describe it and the examiner must use judgement to rate its presence.

16.003 Dulled perception

This symptom is the opposite of 'heightened perception' (item **16.004**). Those affected experience their environment as dark or grey, uniform and uninteresting and flat. Tastes and appetites are blunted, colors may appear to be muddy and dirty, sounds to be ugly or impure. Once the symptom has disappeared it may be difficult to remember or describe and the examiner must use judgement to rate its presence.

Differentiation from other symptoms:

The symptom should be rated present only when there is a definite perceptual change, e.g. lack of interest would not qualify.

16.004 Heightened perception

Sounds seem unnaturally clear or loud or intense, colors appear more brilliant or beautiful, details of the environment seem to stand out in a particularly interesting way, and any sensation may be experienced exceptionally vividly. The pattern on a wallpaper, or the cracks in a ceiling, may become insistently noticeable. Once the symptom has disappeared, the respondent often finds it difficult to remember or describe, and the examiner must use judgement to rate its presence.

16.005 Changed perception of time

The subject's perception of time seems to change, so that it appears to flow very slowly or very rapidly or to change its tempo. Time may appear to stop altogether. Include the experience that events appear to happen exactly as they happened before, so that the subject feels that he has relived them exactly (deja vu), and the experience that common events are completely new, as though they had never happened before. Once such symptoms have disappeared it may be difficult for the subject to remember or describe it and the examiner must use judgement to rate its presence.

Differentiation from other symptoms:

Depressed patients often feel that time has become viscous, that it hangs heavy, although when they look back over a period it seems to have passed quickly. It is sometimes difficult to differentiate this description from boredom. Manic patients, by contrast, are particularly prone to sensing the passage of time as effortlessly flowing. Very strange abnormalities of time perception are sometimes seen in schizophrenia - it may suddenly seem to stop completely and then start again, or its rate may change frequently in an unpredictable way. Rate the experience on its own merits irrespective of possible diagnoses.

16.006 Derealization (things)

In derealization, the emotional component is detached from perception so that respondents experience their surroundings as unreal. The experience has an 'as if' quality. An office or a bus or a street seems as though it is a stage set. Everything seems colorless, artificial and dead.

Differentiation from other symptoms:

Sometimes experiences that sound somewhat like derealization do not have its 'as if' quality and are clearly delusional. These should be rated at item **16.013 / 19.032**.

Distinguish from item **16.003**, 'Dulled Perception', in which there is a physical greyness or lack of color.

16.007 Derealization (People)

The detachment of emotion from perception can apply also to other people. R cannot register the affective drive suggested by the actions of others, so that they seem to be actors, rather than real people going about their ordinary business. They seem to be pretending to have motivations and feelings. In more extreme forms, respondents feel as though people are 'puppets on a string without any real life of their own'. This is an 'as if' phenomenon stemming from the emotional quality of the perception of people. Delusional forms should be rated at item **16.013 / 19.032**.

16.008 Depersonalization

There is a loss of the emotional component of the consciousness of self. The symptom is an 'as if' feeling of the self being unreal, acting a part instead of being spontaneous and natural, a sham, a shadow of a real person. There is a measure of understanding and respondents know the condition is abnormal. They feel detached from their experiences, as though viewing them from a long way off, or through the wrong end of a telescope.

A more severe form of the symptom occurs when respondents feel as if they were actually dead or living an entirely different 'parallel world' and cannot interact in this one. Derealization (items **16.006** and **16.007**) is often present at the same time and should be rated independently.

Sometimes experiences that sound like depersonalization lack its essential 'as if' quality and are clearly delusional. These should be rated under item **16.013 / 19.032**.

16.009 Depersonalized perception of self

This experience is a form of depersonalization. Looking at themselves in a mirror or a photograph, respondents lack the emotional component of self recognition, and feel as if the person represented has no connection with them. They may feel they cannot see a proper reflection.

The delusional form, in which respondents are convinced that they do not exist, or have no thoughts or no mind, is rated at **16.013 / 19.032**.

16.010 Unfamiliarity (self)

This is an extension of **16.009**, in which subjects lack the emotional process by which they recognize parts of their body as being part of themselves. This may be a failure of visual perception or of proprioception or both. They look at part of themselves and feel as if the part does not belong to them.

In delusional forms (rated at **16.013 / 19.032**) they may be convinced, for example, they may say, for example, that they have no head. This symptom is distinguished from the somewhat similar experience of anosognosia, occasioned by neurological malfunction, in which the affected people deny that the limb or other part of the body has anything to do with them.

16.011 Dysmorphophobia

Those affected feel that something has changed about their appearance. The nose is too large, the mouth awry, the teeth too prominent, etc. They acknowledge however that other people cannot see the change and that the feeling is abnormal, although they cannot dispel it for very long. The delusional form is rated at item **16.012**.

16.012 Delusions concerning appearance

See definition of delusions at the beginning of Section 19, and the content of item **16.011**. This delusion is often monothematic (see also item **19.034** in SCAN text).

16.013 Delusions of depersonalization or derealization.

Several earlier symptoms (items **16.006 - 16.010**) have delusional forms that should be rated at this item. In the most extreme form there is a conviction of non - existence (delusion of Cotard). Include delusion that part of the body or mind is missing or not real, and delusions of derealization. See definition of delusions at the beginning of Section 19.

16.014 Other perceptual abnormalities

16.015 Dates of PERIOD/S rated at Section 16

16.016 Rate interference due to Section 16 symptoms

16.017 - 16.018 Identify the organic cause of Section 16 symptoms

Rate whether an 'organic' cause is present here and in Section 20 at items **16.017** and **20.061**, whether or not it can be specified in terms of an ICD - 10 class.

A range of organic conditions (for example, cerebral tumors, temporal lobe epilepsy and other pathologies) can be associated with hallucinations. These can be indicated for individual items by use of the etiology scale and option, or can be attributed for the entire section of item as below. The letter identifying the ICD - 10 chapter, and up to three digits, should be entered at items **16.018, 20.077, 20.079** and **20.081**. A list of ICD - 10 categories is provided in the Appendix.

Psychoactive substances rated in Sections 11 and 12, such as alcohol, cocaine, and amphetamines, which can be associated with hallucinations should be rated in Sections 11 or 12. For example, alcoholic hallucinosis is attributed at item **11.019**, not here. However, individual items can have specific etiologic attribution indicated by use of the etiology scale and option.

Dementias and delirium and other cognitive disorders are rated in Section 21.

17 Hallucinations

GENERAL POINTS ABOUT SECTION 17

Respondents are usually able and willing to describe their experiences and it may be possible to rate many items in this Section without using the specific probes. A bare answer of 'Yes' to a probe is not sufficient for a positive rating. The interviewer must be sure that the respondent has described the relevant experience in his or her own words.

The following general points should be read in conjunction with those for Sections 16, 18 and 19.

Hallucinations are false perceptions. Although usually differentiated from illusions, which are transpositions or distortions of real perceptions, hallucinations may sometimes appear to originate in such a way. For example, a respondent may describe voices that only speak when a bird cries. What matters in rating relevant PSE10 items is whether the experience fits the relevant item definition. Similarly, no use is made in this Glossary of the term 'pseudo - hallucination', though there is an item for rating whether hallucinations are experienced entirely in the mind or as originating outside it. Even here, however, the break in continuity is somewhat artificial. Voices may be experienced as 'in the mind', in the head, in the ears, in the throat (perhaps substituted for the Respondent's voice), on the surface of the body or at any distance from it.

A few items (**17.023, 17.025, 17.027, 17.029**) are concerned with delusions that are based on hallucinations and difficult to separate from them. They are 'secondary' elaborations or interpretations. See the beginning of Section 19.

Differentiation from other symptoms:

These characteristics distinguish hallucinations from Section 16 experiences and from vivid imagery (e.g. eidetic imagery).

17.001 Probe for hallucinations

An exploratory probe, which is asked only if there has been no indication earlier in the interview that hallucinations are present. The rating is not used in algorithms except as a cut - off.

17.002 Probe for other unusual perceptual experiences

All forms of unusual odd or unpleasant experiences, not explicable in terms of practices sanctioned as normal within a recognized social group, should be included under this heading; for example, odd beliefs, magical or extra-sensory powers such as telepathy or clairvoyance, superstitions that go well beyond those common in the local community.

This probe might elicit other forms of hallucination which should be included at item **17.001.**

Proceed beyond the cut - off point if there is any doubt.

AUDITORY HALLUCINATIONS

17.003 Nonverbal auditory hallucinations

This symptom includes noises, other than words, which have no real origin in the world outside, and no explicable origin in bodily processes, which respondents regard as separate from their own mental processes. Thus tinnitus or the sound of the subject's heart beating are not included, nor is the memory of a piece of music. Consciousness is clear. Any auditory hallucinations taking the form of recognizable words are excluded.

Rate, for example, noises such as music, tapping, birds' cries, hissing, etc., if clearly not occurring in reality and not part of the individual's memories or voluntary imaginings. Include if whispering, muttering or mumbling is heard but no words are intelligible. (But include if R 'knows' what is being 'said' by the noise, without hearing any words). If there are recognizable words as well rate onc or more of the other symptoms concerning auditory hallucinations in preference.

17.004 Frequency of verbal auditory hallucinations

The item is self - explanatory.

17.005 Length of utterances

The item is self - explanatory. Include here voices that are of a derogatory or threatening nature (rating 4).

17.006 Quality of auditory hallucinations

'Voices' may sound distorted, or have a quality that distinguishes them from real ones. Rate (1) if this is so; rate (2) if the voices have the quality of real voices.

17.007 Internal hallucinations

Inner voices or images, perceived with the vividness and concreteness characteristic of hallucinations but lacking external projection. When asked to describe them, R may localize them as occurring 'within the mind' or 'within the head' but they cannot readily be provoked or altered at will. The lack of projection into external, objective space is not 'insight', which may or may not be present (see item **17.013**). Confusion should not occur between the space of the body and the mind as they may not overlap and may not be identical. Voices that occur in the mind must be therefore separated from those occurring outside the mind.

Such symptoms(i.e. voices occurring in the mind) are often termed 'pseudo - hallucinations', but this term can be used in other ways.

17.008 Voices commenting on thoughts or actions

A voice or voices speaking about respondents and therefore referring to them in the third person. Consciousness is clear. The content is not congruent with depressive or elated mood. (Exclude for example, '*This man is evil, we must hang him*', in a context of depressed mood.)

Rate if the voice is heard commenting on thoughts or actions in the third person, or if voices talk to each other about the respondent.

Differentiation from other symptoms:

Be careful to distinguish the symptom from delusions of reference (items **19.004 - 19.006**), in which respondents say that other people talk about them, usually disparagingly. This may be a delusional inference from apparently meaningful glances from people talking amongst themselves at a distance, and thus be described in similar terms to an hallucination. Or a murmur of voices from people talking among themselves may be misinterpreted as a derogatory remark. If in doubt, rate (8).

17.009 Second and third person auditory hallucinations

This item evaluates the relative prominence of second and third person auditory hallucinations. Second person 'voices' are heard speaking directly to the respondent. Consciousness is clear. The tone and content of the voices may be pleasant and supportive, neutral or hostile, threatening or accusatory.

Third person voices are experienced as speaking about R, often between themselves.

Differentiation from other symptoms:

Do not include voices saying one or two words only, unless it is clear from other information that R is understating the length of hallucinatory utterances. Very brief comments can be rated (1) at item **17.005**.

Be careful to distinguish the symptom from delusions of reference, items **19.004 - 19.006**. (See differential definition at item **17.008** above.)

17.010 Congruence of auditory hallucinations with affective state

This item is identical with that at **6.021**. If a different rating is entered here it will be used in preference to the earlier one.

Auditory hallucinations may be congruent with an affective state when there is a clear pathological mood of depression or elation and the content is clearly appropriate to the mood.

In the case of depressed mood, the content is deprecatory or consistent with depressive delusional ideas (e.g. 'You are sinful', 'It is the job of the police to deal with criminals like you'). Sometimes nonverbal auditory hallucinations can be mood congruent, as in the example of depressed patients who hear the sounds of gallows being erected outside their hospital rooms.

In the case of elated mood the content must likewise be grandiose or related to manic delusions (e.g. 'Go to the palace, they will make you king').

Be careful to distinguish this symptom from delusions of reference consistent with affective disturbance (items **19.010** and **19.011**) in which respondents think that other people talk about them but are misinterpreting murmurs from their conversation or what they think are meaningful glances. Illusions, as when subjects think they hear their name called in a crowd, should be excluded.

In other words the use of this item implies that there is a preexisting mood change that is pervasive against a background of which the congruence of the psychotic experiences are being assessed. Rate based upon the understandability of the psychotic experiences in the light of the patient's overall psychopathology.

17.011 Mood rated congruent at item 17.010

The item is self - explanatory.

17.012 Special features of auditory hallucinations

A number of unusual characteristics of auditory hallucinations may be rated here. One is the phenomenon known as 'functional' hallucination, where the hallucination is only apparent through another, real, noise. So for example subjects may experience auditory hallucinations only while a tap is running - the hallucination starts when the tap is turned on and ceases when it is turned off. Note that the individual perceives both the hallucination and the real experience. Also include here hallucinations that seem to come from part of the respondent's body. If the hallucinatory voice appears to originate from the mouth, be careful to distinguish from item **18.013**, replaced control of R's own voice.

17.013 Insight into auditory hallucinations

The respondent's explanation of the phenomena described is rated in terms of its content. Note that patients may have insight into their illness without having insight into their perceptual anomalies. In other words, rate here respondent's insight into the percept per se and not the illness in general.

17.014 Prominence of auditory hallucinations

Consider intrusiveness; loudness, persistence, frequency, and interference with mental functions. A rating of (3) means that hallucinations are the central feature of the clinical picture during the period rated. A rating of (2) means that other symptoms (delusions, affective symptoms, etc.) are equally prominent. A rating of (1) means that hallucinations are not intrusive, frequent or persistent compared with other symptoms.

VISUAL HALLUCINATIONS

The subsection begins with a set of probes intended to elicit a description of the nature and content of R's experiences.

R sees objects, people, images that other people cannot see. Consciousness is clear (except in the case of hallucinations associated with waking or going to sleep). The vision may appear to be in the external world or within the R's own mind. Organic causes and drug effects should be rated in Sections 11, 12 and 21.

17.015   Unformed visual hallucinations

The subject sees formless images, flashes, shadows, colored lights, in clear consciousness. Distinguish however from misinterpretations of real stimuli (such as an anxious person thinking there is an intruder in the shadows).

17.016   Formed visual hallucinations

The subject sees particular objects or people superimposed on the real visual field, in clear consciousness. Be careful to exclude phenomena of this type that appear during temporal lobe ictus.

17.017   Scenic visual hallucinations

Under this item are rated hallucinatory experience which comprise more than single specific objects. The person afflicted sees whole scenes largely or completely replacing the actual content of the visual field. Consciousness must be clear, and the interviewer must be aware that scenic visual hallucinations are a fairly common feature of temporal lobe epilepsy. However, they do occur in functional psychoses of all kinds. One person, for example, saw visions of hellfire complete with devils when he was depressed, and Christ surrounded by choirs of angels when he was elated.

17.018   Hypnogogic and hypnopompic hallucinations

Hypnogogic hallucinations may be auditory or visual or both. Occasionally they involve other modalities. They occur during the period of falling to sleep; hypnopompic hallucinations during the corresponding period of waking. Respondents may claim that they are fully awake when this is not the case. For this reason, hallucinations experienced during a time of probable drowsiness should not be rated positive at items **17.015 - 17.017** unless it is certain that consciousness is clear. The hallucinations are not continuous. Respondents do not participate in them as in a dream. The content of visual hallucinations may be abstract shapes, faces, figures, scenes from nature. Auditory hallucinations include animal noises, music or voices, particularly a voice calling the subject's name.

These hallucinations are common in normal subjects, particularly after sleep deprivation, but also occur in clinical disorders.

OTHER HALLUCINATIONS

17.019   Hallucinations associated with bereavement

Visual hallucinations are not uncommon following bereavement or other forms of personal loss. Those affected see the lost person in a characteristic situation, sitting in a chair or working in the kitchen or garden. Such experiences are often associated with hearing the well - known voice, saying some familiar phrase, or hearing familiar movements in one of the rooms. The experience may only involve a voice, without any visual content. Include all forms of these hallucinations in the rating. The experience is usually fleeting.

17.020   Dissociative hallucinations

The typical example is of someone who can see, and/or engage in an active two-way conversation with, another, usually well - known, person. Other modalities (touch, smell, etc.) may also be involved. Such episodes can vary in length from very brief to an hour or so.

Dissociative hallucinations sometimes occur in the context of special religious or subculturally accepted practices, as when the respondent is a member of a cult or family with such beliefs and practices. Films, television programs or books may be another influence. These hallucinations always occur in a background of dissociation.

If dissociative phenomena are suspected, items **2.053 - 2.070** should be considered.

Differentiation from other symptoms:

Similar experiences can occur in a variety of disorders though usually in a more passive mode. Two - way conversations can sometimes be inferred from the content of 'replies' spoken by people who have no dissociative symptoms, though the hallucinations are rarely multimodal. However, any supposedly underlying disorder should not be taken into account when making the rating. Temporal lobe epilepsy and intracranial tumor should be considered.

17.021   Prominence of VH in total clinical picture

Use the same criteria as for item **17.014**.

17.022   Olfactory hallucinations

Simple olfactory hallucinations, such as a smell of orange peel or perfume, or a smell of 'death' or burning, which other people cannot smell, are rated here. Be sure that there is no more obvious cause such as sinusitis, or misinterpretation of a smell that really is present. If the experience is delusionally elaborated, rate item **17.023**.

If subjects think that they themselves smell, rate item **17.024**, while a delusion that others think that R smells is rated at item **17.025**.

17.023 Delusions associated with smell

In this case, there often, though not always, appears to be an olfactory hallucination, but this is elaborated in delusional terms. One woman not only smelled gas, but believed it was being piped into her room by the neighbor above. Another thought that a chemical smell she could detect was evidence that there was a bomb factory next door. Delusions associated with real smells should also be rated here.

17.024 Hallucination that R gives off a smell

Under this item, subjects adhere more or less strongly to the belief that they give off a smell that can be detected by others. This smell is almost always described as unpleasant and may lead to considerable social withdrawal. The symptom sometimes occurs in severe depressive conditions, but also constitutes the basis of the so called olfactory paranoid syndrome, one of the monothematic delusional states. If the latter, remember to rate item **19.034**. The essence of the symptom lies in the self-reference - the subject gives off a smell that others notice in an adverse way.

17.025 Delusion that others think R smells

This item is placed with the hallucinations for convenience of interviewing. It concerns a delusion (usually monothematic, although the theme is often pervasive in the sense that it affects many fields of attitude and action) that other people are thinking or saying that R gives off a smell.

17.026 Sexual hallucinations

Hallucinations of the kind described at item **17.027** are rarely described without delusional elaboration or explanation and should usually be rated there. Rate here only if the interviewer is satisfied that the experience is truly hallucinatory and not vivid self stimulating fantasy.

17.027 Delusions associated with sexual hallucinations

A range of delusions may be based on interpretations and elaborations of sexual hallucinations. Respondents may say that ghosts make love to them as they lie in bed, or that they experience sexual arousal as a result of alien influence, perhaps induced by telepathy. Rate only the delusion, not the hallucination. Include also a delusion that R's sex is changing, or that R is pregnant.

17.028 Hallucinations of other senses

Hallucinations other than those described above tend to be described in unusual terms and lack explanation in those terms. For example, respondents may claim they are being touched at times when there is no-one or nothing around to do the touching. Others may complain of sudden sensations of heat, or pain, or crawling sensations. Food may taste burnt or acid. There may be feelings of floating.

Differentiation from other symptoms:

The interviewer should consider paresthesias associated with neurological disorder and 'formication', the sensation of insects crawling over the body, which can result from intoxication, particularly with cocaine. The former should be excluded, the latter rated at item **12.043.4**.

17.029 Bizarre delusions apparently associated with bodily sensations

Delusional elaborations of items rated at **17.028**. Such elaborations are often couched in bizarre terms. Respondents may claim to being subjected to torture, that they have ice instead of a heart, that they have been caused to float in the air, that their organs are misplaced or their liver turned to gold.

Hallucinations of taste may be interpreted in terms of food being deliberately poisoned, although in some cases this is a persecutory delusion (item **19.012**) without a primary change in taste. Tactile hallucinations may be associated with delusional interpretations of infestation by insects or other parasites.

Rate here also the symptom of somatic passivity.

17.030 Apparent hallucinatory experiences NOS

17.031 Age at first onset of hallucinations

17.032 Date/s of PERIOD/S of Section 17 symptoms

17.033 Interference due to Section 17 symptoms

17.034 Organic cause of Section 17 symptoms

A simple rating of whether an 'organic' cause is present, whether or not it can be specified in terms of an ICD-10 class can be recorded at **17.034** and in Section 20 at items **20.062, 20.063,** and **20.064.** Four general rules are used to make such attributions of cause and are set out in Section 13 of the Glossary:

17.035 Identify the organic cause of Section 17 symptoms

A range of organic conditions (for example, cerebral tumors, temporal lobe epilepsy and other pathologies) can be associated with hallucinations. These can be indicated for individual items by use of the etiology scale and option, or can be attributed for the entire section of item as below. The letter identifying the ICD - 10 chapter, and up to three digits, should be entered at items **17.035, 20.077, 20.079** or **20.081**. A list of ICD - 10 categories is provided in the Appendix.

Psychoactive substances rated in Sections 11 and 12, such as alcohol, cocaine, and amphetamines, which can be associated with hallucinations should also be rated in Sections 11 or 12. For example, alcoholic hallucinosis is attributed at item **11.019**. However, individual items can have specific etiologic attribution indicated by use of the etiology scale and option.

Dementias and delirium and other cognitive disorders are rated in Section 21.

18 Subjectively described thought disorder and experience of replacement of will

GENERAL POINTS ABOUT SECTION 18

The following general points should be read in conjunction with those for Sections 16, 17 and 19.

It is easy to record many Section 18 symptoms as present on inadequate evidence because respondents may answer affirmatively without having understood the questions. If interviewers, too, do not have the specific definitions in mind, and lead R without cross - examination, errors are likely to occur.

Particular care is necessary when respondents have a language or speech problem of any kind (see Section 15). They must be able to give a clear description of the symptom. A response of 'Yes' to a question, in itself, provides no evidence either way.

Item **18.001** is placed first for convenience of interviewing, since it deals with an abnormal primary experience that often leads to delusion formation (see the beginning of Section 19). Item **18.002** is a probe for experiences typical of the Section. Item **18.003** is concerned with a delusion that is sometimes confused with later Section 18 items. It provides an opportunity to clarify the phenomenology at an early stage.

Several other confusing problems, potentially capable of leading to false positive ratings of many Section 18 symptoms, should be kept in mind. Those involving subjectively described thought disorder are described at items **18.004 - 18.011**. Those involving the experience of replacement of will (items **18.012 - 18.017**) are described after item **18.011**. Some more general points are made below.

(1) Some respondents, because of an inadequate intellectual level or language problems rated in Section 15, are unable to grasp what is being asked, or to give a rateable answer. In such cases, do not give the benefit of the doubt. Make full use of a rating of (8), if there is some possibility that the symptom has not been excluded, or (9), if it is impossible to tell.

(2) Symptoms such as obsessions (Section 5), loss of concentration (item **7.002**), inefficient thinking (item **7.003**), and ideomotor pressure (item **10.004**), may lead respondents who experience them to give affirmative answers to questions about Section 18 symptoms. The interviewer should have no difficulty, however, since none of these symptoms involve alien thoughts experienced as being inserted into the mind or any of the other specific features given in the definitions below.

(3) Voices experienced as being within the mind may be difficult to distinguish from Section 18 symptoms since respondents are sometimes unable to say whether the

experience is a voice or a thought. In such cases rate both symptoms as present. If the experience is of 'loud thoughts', rate item **18.004**.

(4) The respondent may experience thought insertion and explain it in delusional terms (e.g. as due to hypnotism or telepathy). In such a case both types of symptoms are present. However, a statement that the respondent is being subjected to telepathy, being hypnotised, being influenced, or simply that thoughts are being read, rate the appropriate items but not Section 18 symptoms (except **18.003**). A delusion of influence is often not based on thought insertion. Similarly, delusions of religious influence are not necessarily based on thought insertion. Although the content of thinking is influenced by God or the Devil, etc. the thoughts themselves are R's. In other words do not rate only explanatory delusions.

(5) An elated individual may speak as if thoughts were coming from elsewhere, e.g. they are so magnificent that it seems as if they must have come from the sun, so good that they must have come from God, etc. But in such cases the thoughts belong to R, although they may be ascribed to God in the sense that their source is God.

18.001 Delusional mood and perplexity

Respondents feel that familiar surroundings have changed in a way that may be difficult to describe but that is charged with significance and self - reference and, above all, puzzling. Something odd seems to be going on and the atmosphere may rapidly seem to become ominous and threatening. R seeks for an explanation, which may be based on misinterpretations of ordinary observations or on perceptual abnormalities. This part of the episode often ends abruptly, with the formation of hallucinations or delusions.

Differentiation from other symptoms:

Some respondents agree with the probe when all they mean is that unexpected things often happen.

Care must be taken to differentiate the symptom from derealization or depersonalization (items **16.006 - 16.009**).

People with expansive mood (item **10.001**) often have a heightened sense of the meaning of their surroundings and objects may take on a special significance. The development of the process is congruent with the mood, which is the central feature. Moreover, the experience is exalting rather than threatening, and oceanic rather than self referential. However, the symptom should be rated on its own merits.

18.002 Probe for Section 18 symptoms

This general probe should become more specific if there is any reason to suppose that the symptom might be present. However, the general point made about probes for hallucinations holds with the same force for Section 18 symptoms. These experiences must not be rated as present simply on the basis of the respondent's assent to a leading question. The experience must be described in R's own words.

18.003 Delusion that thoughts are being read

This is usually an explanatory delusion. Often it goes with delusions of reference or misinterpretation, which require some explanation of how other people know so much about R's future movements. It may be an elaboration of thought broadcast, thought insertion, auditory hallucinations, delusions of control, delusions of persecution or delusions of influence. It can occur with expansive delusions (e.g. when R wishes to explain how Einstein stole his original ideas). The symptom should not be mistaken for symptoms such as thought insertion or broadcast.

18.004 Loud thoughts

Respondents say that their own thoughts seem to sound 'aloud' in their head, almost as though someone standing nearby could hear them. Respondents recognize that thinking, which is normally a silent process, is now taking the form of sound.

Differentiation from other symptoms:

If thoughts are repeated, rate at item **18.005**. It may sometimes require care to distinguish the symptom from auditory hallucinations, where respondents no longer experience the loud thoughts as their own. Hallucinations of voices repeating R's thoughts are rated at item **17.008**. Thought echo has its own item **18.005** and is not included here. Obsessional ruminations may sometimes be considered but the experience of loud thoughts should only be rated after a clear description; ruminations are seldom that.

18.005 Thought echo

This item is often rated positively on insufficient evidence. Respondents experience their own thoughts as repeated or echoed (not spoken aloud, item **18.004**) with very little interval between the original and the echo. The repetition may not be perfect, however, but subtly or grossly changed in quality.

Differentiation from other symptoms:

Distinguish from auditory hallucinations of voices repeating R's thoughts (item **17.008**).

18.006 Thought insertion

The essence of the item is that respondents lack the normal sense of ownership of the thoughts in their mind. Their thoughts are experienced as alien, not their own. The symptom excludes a belief that R has unwanted thoughts; for example, if the Devil seems to be inducing evil thoughts. In the most typical case, the alien thoughts are said to have been inserted into the mind from outside, by means of radar or telepathy or some other means. In such a case there is an explanatory delusion as well (e.g. items **19.021 - 19.023**). However, a positive rating does not depend upon the presence of an explanatory delusion; nor are delusions of telepathy, hypnotism, etc., necessarily based on thought insertion.

Sometimes respondents may say they do not know where the alien thoughts came from, although they are quite clear that they are not their own. In very rare instances, they may postulate that they come from the unconscious mind - while still consciously experiencing them as alien. These experiences are included in the symptom.

18.007 Thought 'broadcast'

This item is often rated positively on insufficient evidence. The essence of the symptom is that respondents experience their thoughts as diffusing out of their minds so that they can be experienced by others. The term 'broadcast' should not be misunderstood. The experience is passive, in the sense that it is not willed but experienced. Moreover, there is no necessary implication that the thoughts can be heard. Thus thinking which is normally a private experience no longer remains so.

Differentiation from other symptoms:

Any mechanism put forward by R to explain the experience of thought insertion is rated independently.

A belief in the ability to transmit thoughts to others should not be rated as thought broadcast. It is a delusion of grandiose ability (**10.016 / 19.029**).

The symptom is a rare one. Distinguish it from thought reading. Respondents often say that their thoughts are being read, without having had the experience of thought broadcast. What they mean is that other people can tell from their expression, or from their habits, what they are likely to be thinking. Thought reading can also be an explanatory delusion. For example, if respondents have an extensive system of delusions of reference so that wherever they go they seem to be followed, or people are making signs at them, they may say that whoever is organizing it can read their thoughts, thus knowing where they are going to go and how to instruct others to react. 'Thought broadcast' is only rated when R actually experiences thoughts being available to others.

Distinguish from internal hallucinations (**17.007**) in which respondents hear voices within their minds, not coming from outside. The voice is distinguishable from R's own thoughts.

Distinguish also from thought withdrawal (item **18.010**) in which thoughts are not experienced as broadcast or shared, but as withdrawn so that subjects have no thoughts.

18.008 Thought commentary

R reports that there is more than one stream of thought in the mind. Thoughts recognized as alien or intruded may comment on R's thoughts or on something R is doing or reading or writing.

Differentiation from other symptoms:

This is not the same as a hallucinatory voice doing the same thing (rate **17.008**), though it may, of course, be a precursor.

18.009 Thought block

Thought block is rare and should only be rated present when the examiner is quite sure that it is. If there is any doubt, it is probably not present. While they are flowing freely R experiences a sudden and unexpected stopping of thought. When this occurs it is dramatic and usually happens on several occasions. The experience is passive.

Differentiation from other symptoms:

The passivity distinguishes the symptom from the common experience of losing a train of thought, which is often associated with anxiety (e.g. 'exam nerves'), or with distraction, when respondents are searching actively for their thoughts.

Distinguish from the somewhat similar delusion of depersonalization (item **16.013 / 19.032**) in which there is a complaint of having no thoughts in the mind, but not that thoughts have suddenly stopped.

18.010 Thought withdrawal

Although R may be unable to describe pure thought block, it is recognizable when it is expressed in terms of thought withdrawal. Respondents say that their thoughts have been taken out of their minds so that they have no thoughts. The experience is passive in the same sense as that of thought broadcast (item **18.007**); it is not willed but experienced. The difference is that no thoughts are left behind and there is an experience of actual withdrawal which often leads to explanatory delusions.

18.011 Other subjective disorder of thought

Include other manifestations of the basic experience. For example respondents may report that their thoughts are moved from left to right, that they cannot tell which are their own thoughts, that they sense their thoughts as outside their head. Note that the last example is not the same as thought withdrawal.

GENERAL POINTS ITEMS 18.012 - 18.017: EXPERIENCE OF REPLACEMENT OF WILL

The essential element in definition is that respondents experience their will as replaced by the intentions of some other force or agency. The experience is passive, in that it is not under conscious control, but it may be actively resented.

The basic experience may be elaborated in various ways - respondents believe that someone else's words are coming out using their voice, or that what they write is not their own, or that they are the victim of possession - a zombie or a robot controlled by someone else's will, even their bodily movements being willed by some other power.

Differentiation from other symptoms:

Respondents must be able to understand the probes and give a clear description of the symptom. A response of 'Yes' to a probe, provides no evidence, in itself, as to its presence or absence. The presence of any language problems rated in Section 15 necessitates particular caution. Unless the examiner is confident that respondents have indeed had this experience, the symptom is probably absent. When in doubt, rate (8), (9) or (0) according to circumstances.

A statement that some physical or supernatural force is 'controlling' or 'influencing' the respondent, without a description of the basic experience is not sufficient to make a positive rating. Respondents may mean only that their life is planned and directed by fate or that the future is already present in embryo, or that they are not very strong-willed in the face of pressures and demands from those they mix with. Respondents may mean that voices are giving them orders; that God is omnipotent and controls everything including them, or that they themselves are God (this is a religious delusion, item **19.021**). Such responses can only be rated in Section 18 if the essential element of all the constituent symptoms is present, namely that the feeling of personal intention has been replaced by a sense that some other will is in control.

The experience is not based on mood change. If the description appears to be an explanation or elaboration of symptoms based on mood change, Section 18 items are rated (0).

For example, do not include the statement of an elated subject who says that God is controlling his or her personal actions. Far from the will being replaced, it is greatly strengthened, as if it were God's.

If R describes a socially shared experience, or one which is explicable in terms of a prolongation of a socially sanctioned experience, rate item **2.057 - 2.059**. If purely cultural, no symptom is rateable. For example, a Taoist priestess who said that she was controlled by the God when she was in a trance, would not be rated on this ground alone as having any Section 18 symptom. Nor would spiritualists, or respondents whose motivation is more specifically personal, as when Mozart is said to be dictating his music to R from beyond the grave. (Consider dissociative symptoms, e.g. item **17.020** and items **2.057 - 2.059**.)

18.012 Replacement of will by external force

The general definition given above is directly applicable to this item, which deals with the experience in pure form.

18.013 Replaced control of voice

Respondents feel that their voice is under the control of an outside agency and produce speech without a sense of intention. They may be surprised by what they say or by the odd quality of their voice, which may be difficult to accept as their own.

18.014 Replaced control of handwriting

Respondents feel that the movements and content of their handwriting or typing are alien, not intended by them, not under their control, taken over by an outside force or agency. Exclude statements that suggest dissociative mechanisms such as the example of taking dictation from well - known historical figures.

18.015 Replaced control of actions

A similar alienation to that of item **18.014** but involving any other actions, for example walking or running. In extreme cases, respondents may feel that nothing they do is the product of their intentions.

18.016 Replaced control of affect

This can be seen as a form of an alienation experience where the respondent experiences that his/her emotions are not under his/her volitional control but under the influence of an alien will.

18.017 Other types of replaced control

Other experiences include 'made' impulses invoking actual actions (as in **18.015**), i.e. respondents feel that they have an urge to do something which they recognize as not their own.

18.018 Age at first onset of Section 18 symptoms

Enter approximate age if necessary (say, within 5 years or so), since this is more useful than leaving the boxes blank.

18.019 Date/s of PERIOD/S of Section 18 symptoms

18.020 Interference due to Section 18 symptoms

18.021 Organic cause of Section 18 symptoms

Items **18.021, 20.065** and **20.066** allows a simple rating of whether an 'organic' cause is present, whether or not it can be specified in terms of an ICD-10 class.

18.022 Identify the organic cause of Section 18 symptoms

A range of organic conditions (for example, cerebral tumors, temporal lobe epilepsy, Huntington's disease and other pathologies) can be associated with Section 18 symptoms. Individual items can be rated using the etiology scale and option, or the entire section can be attributed to an organic cause below. The letter identifying the ICD-10 chapter, and up to three digits, should be entered at items **18.022, 20.077, 20.079** or **20.081**. A list of ICD-10 categories is provided in the Appendix.

Psychoactive substances rated in Sections 11 and 12, such as alcohol, cocaine, and amphetamines, which can be associated with the symptoms should also be rated in Sections 11 or 12, but can also be indicated for individual items by use of the etiology scale and option.

Dementias and delirium and other cognitive disorders are rated in Section 21.

19 Delusions

The following general points should be read in conjunction with those for 'psychotic' symptoms rated in Sections 16, 17 and 18.

Particular care is necessary when respondents have a language or speech problem of any kind (see Section 15). Vague or rambling answers should be rated under speech disorder. R must be able to give a clear description of the symptom. A response of 'Yes' to a question, in itself, provides no evidence either way.

FOUR NECESSARY BUT NOT SUFFICIENT CHARACTERISTICS OF A DELUSION

(1) The belief is described clearly in the respondent's own words, not simply assented to following a leading question.

(2) It is held with a basic and compelling subjective conviction, though the degree of certainty may fluctuate or be concealed.

(3) It is not susceptible, or only briefly, to modification by experience or evidence that contradict it; i.e. it is incorrigible.

(4) The belief is impossible, incredible or false.

BELIEFS WITH ALL FOUR CHARACTERISTICS THAT ARE NOT DELUSIONAL

Social, cultural, religious and political beliefs

(5) A belief with all the characteristics listed in (1) - (4) is not necessarily idiosyncratic to the individual who holds it. It may be a normal and unsurprising characteristic of belonging to a particular social group and of sharing its dogmas, tenets and values. In other words, beliefs shared and fully explained by particular religious or political or other social groups are not delusional, no matter how passionately they are held, or how false or bizarre they seem to non - members. Thus if a priestess of a particular cult says that she is possessed, when in a trance, by a god (given a special name in that cult), this is understandable in its social context. It is not evidence for a delusional belief. Similarly, when natural events are said to happen by divine intervention in a way that is accepted by all members of the group, there is no delusion, and there are no items in SCAN that allow them to be rated as such.

Overvalued ideas

(6) Some ideas that are held idiosyncratically, i.e. they are not understandable in terms of membership of a social group, may be understandable in terms of the

circumstances and development of a particular personality. For example, a physicist who has spent a lifetime trying to solve a problem may become convinced of an idiosyncratic answer to it although all competent colleagues provide evidence against it and no - one thinks the solution tenable. Such overvalued ideas are 'eccentric', but they sometimes turn out to be true.

Induced 'delusions'

(7) If R, who has never previously been deluded, begins to express abnormal beliefs that are clearly derived (induced) from someone else with whom R is or has become closely related, rate at items **20.026 - 20.028**. These items include the situation where a group of impressionable people are influenced (and sometimes coerced) in this way.

DELUSIONS BASED ON ABNORMAL AFFECT

(8) Beliefs with the four necessary characteristics, which are held idiosyncratically but are clearly based in an abnormal mood, such as depression or elation, are called 'delusion - like', because they are not in themselves 'primary'. In SCAN, they are rated in Sections 6 and 10, and repeated in Section 19. They include beliefs concerned with sin, destitution, catastrophe and grandeur. Such delusions are called 'congruent' with the underlying mood. Examples are given in the text that follows. They can be analyzed separately from other phenomena.

DELUSIONAL ELABORATIONS OF 'PRIMARY' PHENOMENA

(9) If the beliefs are clearly 'secondary' explanations or elaborations of abnormal subjective experiences, defined strictly according to the criteria laid down in Sections 16, 17 and 18, their idiosyncratic and non - social character is particularly evident. They are rated separately from the primary experiences themselves.

PATHOPLASTIC DELUSIONS

(10) Normal social beliefs or overvalued ideas that meet criteria (1) to (4) may be expressed as pathoplastic forms of the delusions described in paragraphs (8) and (9), and may then meet, and be rated on, the relevant criteria. If the respondent claims to be a member of a recognized group, other members usually recognize those aspects of R's belief that are alien to their own. If the beliefs are expressed in a form that is culturally based and recognized as abnormal, such as 'Koro', 'Latah' or 'Witigo', rate at item **19.024**.

PRIMARY DELUSIONS

(11) Some delusions appear as 'primary' experiences in themselves, in that the content is not understandable in terms of any antecedents such as are specified in paragraphs (5) to (10) above. Item **18.001** (delusional mood or 'atmosphere')

describes a prior experience out of which such a delusion may inexplicably be crystallized. In item **19.009**, 'delusional perception' or 'primary delusion' (the nature of the experience is variously interpreted by experts as cognitive, perceptual, or both), the delusional meaning of an experience or set of experiences becomes manifest, often suddenly or over a short period of time. These two items allow a specific rating of these primary phenomena. Other items, such as many delusions of reference, may originate in this way, but it is not feasible or necessary to try to make the distinction each time an item is rated, any more than it is for delusions arising from other primary phenomena; see paragraph (9).

19.001 - 19.002   Probes for Section 19

These probes are self - explanatory. By this time in the interview the possibility of delusions being present will usually be fairly evident. As usual, continue below the cut - off if there is any doubt.

DELUSIONS OF REFERENCE AND MISINTERPRETATION

Items **19.003 - 19.011** are varieties of delusions of reference. They involve an incorrect attribution of significance to people, objects or events that are perceived normally. Thus they are neither hallucinations nor illusions.

Delusions of this type may take the form of a sudden conviction that a given set of perceptions refers to the respondent and has a special significance (item **19.009**). If this is the case, the delusion of reference should be rated in its own right.

19.003   Delusions of being spied upon

This is a particular form of the delusion of reference in which subjects may believe that they are being followed or otherwise observed, or that what they say or do is being recorded on tape. A not uncommon type involves subjects supposedly seeing the same cars in different locations, with the inference that the occupants are engaged in surveillance.

19.004   Delusions of reference

Ideas of self-reference are rated in items **3.010** and **6.014**. Delusions of reference consist of a further elaboration of this experience in so far as other people are involved. Thus what is said may have a double meaning, or someone makes a gesture which subjects construe as a deliberate message, e.g. someone crossing his legs may be taken to mean that R is homosexual. The whole neighborhood may seem to be gossiping about respondents far beyond the bounds of possibility, or they may see references to themselves on the television or in newspapers. Items **19.005 - 19.011** concern extensions to other situations.

Differentiation from other symptoms:

Be careful to distinguish this symptom from auditory hallucinations. It is, of course, possible for respondents to have both symptoms but they are not identical. If they answer 'Yes' to a question about hearing voices, it may be that they think people are talking about them, or making remarks intended for them to overhear, when they are in their presence. If so, it is most likely that they are misinterpreting, not hearing voices. Careful questioning should enable the examiner to judge whether one or other or both symptoms are present.

19.005 Delusional misinterpretation

This item is a further extension of the delusion of reference in that not only do people seem to refer to R directly but whole situations are interpreted in a self-referential way. The arrangement of objects may seem to have special significance. Things seem to be arranged to test respondents, street signs or advertisements on buses, or patterns of color seem to have been put there in order to give messages. This may go so far that whole armies of people may seem to be preoccupied with R. Delusions of persecution or grandeur or other delusional interpretations may not be present. If they are, rate independently.

19.006 Quotation of ideas

Respondents hear people around them, or someone on the radio or television, say something connected with what they have just been thinking. This symptom should be distinguished from auditory hallucination and from thought broadcast (item **18.007**).

19.007 Delusional misidentification

In this item, although there is no change in perception, respondents misidentify those around them in a way that fits their own self - reference and their overall delusional system. They may claim that bystanders are people from their past brought in, in order to convey some kind of special message to them. They may believe that medical or nursing staff are impostors. This is otherwise known as the Fregoli Syndrome.

19.008 Familiar people impersonated

Respondents believe that people well known to them, often friends or members of the family, are not who they purport to be, but are being deliberately impersonated by strangers. The clinical context can be very varied and the symptom should be rated (as with all PSE items) independently of possible diagnosis (Capgras Syndrome).

19.009 Delusional perception

A delusional perception, or primary delusion, is an intrusive, often sudden, knowledge that a common percept has a radically transformed meaning. A normal percept, image or memory takes on an entirely new significance. The initial perception may sometimes be related to a specific experience that makes the effect more dramatic. For example, someone undergoing liver biopsy felt, as the needle was inserted, that he had been chosen by God. A woman getting off a bus on a November night was struck on the forehead by a leaf and immediately knew she had been sent to save the world. Another woman saw a plane cross the sun and at once knew that alien beings had chosen her for their ambassador on earth. In other cases, the process is more prolonged though it usually has a clear onset in one or a set of percepts.

Differentiation from other symptoms:

The experience may follow a period of delusional perplexity (item **18.001**). Many other delusions may be elaborated from such an experience. Always rate any resulting or explanatory delusions independently.

The delusion cannot be explained in terms of an abnormal affect other than delusional mood, nor of the respondent's cultural and social beliefs. Do not include delusions which seem to arise on the basis of a particular mood (e.g. depressive delusions, or grandiose delusions occurring when the patient is elated). Delusions which are explanations of other phenomena, such as thought insertion, hallucinations, subcultural beliefs, etc. should be rated separately.

19.010   Delusional ideas of reference based on guilt

People suffering from severe depression may believe that others are blaming them for, or accusing them of, actions or feelings about which they themselves feel guilty. One woman thought the local council were leaving 'skips' (containers for the disposal of waste) in her neighborhood, as a hidden message that they knew she had not been keeping up her usual high standards of cleanliness and housework. Another thought that nursing staff were disguised police officers, keeping her under surveillance because of her delusional belief that she had allowed a cannabis plant to grow in her garden.

19.011   Delusional ideas of reference based on expansive mood

Respondents who are elated may have such an expansive notion of their talents, beauty, accomplishments or importance, that they believe they must be the center of admiring attention for the neighborhood.

19.012   Delusions of persecution

Respondents believe that someone, or some organization, or some force or power, is trying to harm them in some way; to damage their reputation, to cause them bodily injury, to drive them mad or to bring about their death.

The symptom may take many forms, from the direct belief that people are hunting them down to complex and often bizarre plots, with every kind of science fiction elaboration.

A simple delusion of reference, e.g. that R is being followed or spied upon, is not included unless R believes that harm is intended, in which case rate both symptoms as present. This item should be rated whether or not it is related to pathological mood states.

Delusionally depressed patients often think they are to be tortured or executed, and elated patients may feel persecuted by those who are not persuaded by their grandiose plans.

19.013 Delusions of conspiracy

These are frequently based on delusions of persecution or reference, but may be based on the experience of thought disorder or other passivity phenomena, or of hallucinations. Elated subjects may believe that people around them are collectively organizing to help them. Rate any delusions of conspiracy here, regardless of context.

19.014 Delusional jealousy

This symptom, with all the characteristics of a delusion, is centered around the theme of infidelity. Those affected are convinced that their sexual partner is unfaithful, and virtually every circumstance, however trivial, is adduced as evidence in support of the belief. Signs that might possibly be interpreted as sexual in nature, however unlikely, are taken as confirmation. They may seek evidence, looking for stray hairs on clothing, suspect entries in diaries, signs of sexual activity in underclothing. They may try to catch their partners out by checking that they are where they say they are. Accusations of infidelity may be bizarre, both in terms of the imagined partner and of the nature of the opportunity.

19.015 Non - delusional jealousy

This item (see item **3.013**) is checked here for convenience. Those affected are preoccupied with thoughts that their sexual partner might be or have been unfaithful. They are torn between a belief in their partner's good faith and in their infidelity. They may occasionally give way to a strong desire to behave in the same way as those with the more severe form of the symptom (item **19.014**) but then are ashamed of the thought and the action.

For obvious reasons the judgement of non - delusional but morbid jealousy is difficult to make, particularly if it is unclear whether the partner is actually unfaithful. Moreover, cultural expectations of 'normal' behavior vary widely. If in doubt, rate (8). Infidelity in the partner does not rule out the symptom if the characteristics are present.

19.016 Delusions of pregnancy

Respondents think they are pregnant although the circumstances make it clear that they cannot possibly be. They may be male, or clearly menopausal, or virgin, or abstinent. One subject was a widow, had not had intercourse for several years, and was well past the menopause, but was convinced that she had been pregnant for two years, after a momentary encounter with a stranger in a lift. Why she thought this incident which, from her description, was completely innocent, could have made her pregnant, never came close to consciousness. The symptom has many of the characteristics of a hypochondriacal delusion. It can be associated with a variety of other psychopathological phenomena, or be monothematic (item **19.034** is then rated in addition), and should be rated independently of the clinical context.

19.017 Delusional lover

Usually an idealized love, often, but not necessarily, with someone thought to be of higher status (de Clerambault syndrome). R may follow and pester the supposed lover. The degree of delusional preoccupation can be as high as in delusional jealousy (item **19.014**).

Differentiation from other symptoms:

Differentiate from sexual delusions associated with hallucinations (item **17.027**). Distinguish from vivid fantasies, into the nature of which R has at least occasional insight.

19.018 Delusion that others accuse R of homosexuality

Respondents who apparently have no particular leaning towards their own sex nevertheless believe that they are being accused of being homosexual. They may think they overhear remarks about some peculiarity of gait or manner or physique, or base their conviction on the interpretation of 'meaningful' looks and signs. The symptom can be associated with a variety of other psychopathological phenomena, or be monothematic, and should be rated independently of the clinical context.

19.019 Delusional memories and fantastic delusions

Delusional memories are experiences of past events which clearly did not occur but which the subject equally clearly remembers, e.g. "*I came down to earth on a silver star in 1964*". "*I can remember the knitting needles when they tried to abort me in my mother's womb*". One man claimed that he could remember walking dryshod from Wales to Ireland because the adjacent coasts had moved together. Classically, these memories come suddenly into the mind and have the characteristic of something forgotten once more recollected. Fantastic delusions, unlike, for example, delusions of reference or persecution, are physical impossibilities, rather than social improbabilities. For example, a man maintained that England's coast was melting, as one of a group of 'science fiction' delusions. Delusional confabulations, in which R spontaneously or following a lead produces a flow of fantastic ideas not previously expressed, should be differentiated from confabulation in compensation for short term memory loss (item **21.031** and **21.082**).

Rate fantastic delusions if the content has not been rated elsewhere (e.g. under delusions of paranormal or physical influence, items **19.022** and **19.023**).

19.020 Preoccupation with previous delusions

Occasionally a respondent is preoccupied, not with current morbid phenomena, but with interpretations of past experiences that are no longer present.

19.021 Religious delusions

These are explanations or elaborations of other delusions or psychotic experiences. Do not include well accepted religious beliefs or experiences. See the introduction to this Section of the Glossary.

19.022 Delusional paranormal explanations

Include any delusional explanation or elaboration of other abnormal experience, such as thought insertion or broadcast or delusions of reference or persecution, in terms of paranormal phenomena. Include explanations in terms of hypnotism, telepathy, magic, witchcraft, etc. Note that using the word telepathy merely to describe a process of thought transfer is not a delusional explanation. If telepathy is used in the sense of explaining a mechanism it may be rated here.

Differentiation from other symptoms:

Exclude ideas which are accepted by a sub-cultural group and derived solely from membership in that group.

19.023 Delusional physical explanations

Include any delusional explanation of other abnormal experiences such as thought insertion or broadcast or delusions of reference or persecution or somatic delusions, in terms of physical processes such as electricity, X - Rays, television, radio or machines of various kind. One man thought that burning sensations in his legs were the result of radiation from a local radio transmission station.

19.024 Specifically named local syndrome

There is discussion as to whether locally recognized syndromes such as Latah, Koro and Witigo are simply versions of familiar psychopathological states with their own individual pathoplastic coloring or whether they are syndromes in their own right. If such syndromes are suspected, it is essential to complete the whole SCAN in addition to any detailed local schedule. In this way, co - morbidity can be investigated. Culture Specific Disorders are discussed in Annex 2 of the ICD - 10 DCR. It is suggested there that most such disorders are non - psychotic disorders. The SCAN text includes reminders to reconsider ratings of anxiety and dissociative disorders in such circumstances.

19.025 Delusions of guilt in context of depression

This symptom is grounded in a depressed mood. Those affected think they have brought ruin to their family by being in their present condition or that their symptoms are a punishment for their wicked incompetence. In a more severe form of the symptom, there is a delusional conviction that they have sinned greatly, or committed some terrible crime, or brought ruin upon the world; i.e. there may be a grandiose quality to the delusion. They may feel that they deserve punishment, even death or hell-fire, because of it. They may say that their offense and the punishment it has merited are unnameable.

Differentiation from other symptoms:

Distinguish from pathological guilt without delusional elaboration, in which subjects are in general aware that the guilt originates within themselves and is exaggerated (item **6.013**).

19.026 Delusions of catastrophe in context of depression

Respondents believe that terrible things are going to happen to their families and others with whom they are connected. Their family, friends and colleagues may be dragged down to financial ruin, and may end up starving or in prison as a result of R's failings. Delusions of poverty should be rated under this rubric. Affect is depressed. The symptom may be more intense, as when the subject has a delusional conviction that the world is about to end, that some enormous catastrophe has occurred or is going to occur, that the world is decayed, dirty and rotten.

19.027 Hypochondriacal delusions in context of depression

This symptom is in many ways similar to item **19.032**, delusions of depersonalization. Respondents feel that their body is unhealthy, rotten or diseased. They can only be reassured for a brief while that this is not the case. In more intense forms of the symptom, there is a delusional conviction of the presence of incurable cancer, or that the bowels are stopped up or rotting away.

Sometimes it is difficult to decide whether the appropriate rating should be at item **19.032** or **19.037**, as when respondents say they are hollow and have no inner existence because their insides have rotted away. In this instance it is legitimate to rate both items positively. In general, when in doubt, rate **19.032** rather than **19.037**.

19.028 Hypochondriacal delusions without depression

This is the same symptom as 'hypochondriacal conviction', rated at item **2.039**. If it is changed, the new rating will be used instead of the earlier one.

Distinguish from delusions about appearance (**16.012**) and delusional explanations of somatic hallucinations (**17.029**).

19.029 Delusions of grandiose abilities

Respondents think they are chosen by some power, or by destiny, for a special mission or purpose, because of their unusual talents. They believe they are able to read people's thoughts, or that they are particularly good at helping others, that they are much cleverer than anyone else, that they have invented machines, composed music, solved mathematical problems, and so on, beyond most people's comprehension.

19.030 Delusions of grandiose identity

Respondents believe they are famous, rich, titled or related to prominent people. They may believe that they are changelings and that their real parents are royalty.

Differentiation from other symptoms:

Do not include a delusional identification with God or a saint or an angel as grandiose - this should be counted as a religious delusion (item **19.021**).

19.031 Delusions concerning appearance

Those afflicted have a strong feeling that something is wrong with their appearance. They are convinced that they look old or ugly or dead, their skin is cracked, their teeth misshapen, their nose too large or their body crooked. Other people do not notice anything specially wrong, but respondents can be reassured only momentarily if at all. There may be only be one particular complaint and there is usually no elaboration of any kind.

Sometimes respondents act on the delusion, e.g. have their teeth out or repeated plastic operations.

Differentiation from other symptoms

Exclude selfconsciousness, concern about real skin disease, etc. See items **16.008 - 16.013** for differentiation from perceptual disorders, and **19.032** from depersonalization, and item **3.010** for simple ideas of reference.

19.032 Delusions of depersonalization

Respondents have the belief that they have no brain, a hollow within their skull, no thoughts in their heads. In more extreme forms of the symptom, they are convinced that they have no head, that they cannot see themselves in the mirror, that they have a shadow but no body, that they do not exist at all.

Differentiation from other symptoms

Exclude delusional elaboration, e.g. that some force or agency has taken over R's mind and body so that R now has another identity and no independent will (items in Section 18).

19.033 - 19.040 General ratings

Differentiate simple elaboration from systematization. The term systematization implies that if the initial premise is granted the rest of the delusion is logically constructed and internally consistent.

The term bizarre implies that a delusion is patently absurd. However, the Respondents' cultural, social, and education context must be considered before making this judgement. For example, if a patient was a member of a cultural or subcultural group believing in black magic, then delusions about being controlled by spells would not be considered bizarre.

19.041 Age at first ever onset of delusions

19.042 Date/s of PERIOD/S of Section 19 symptoms

19.043 Interference due to Section 19 symptoms

19.044 Organic cause of Section 19 symptoms

Section 19 allows a simple rating of whether an 'organic' cause is present at **19.044** and at item **20.067** whether or not it can be specified in terms of an ICD - 10 class.

If the criteria set out in the Glossary are probably but not completely met in the case of Section 19 symptoms, rate (1). If the attribution of physical cause is confirmed by expert investigation, rate (2). Use (8) if uncertain whether organic or not. The default rating is (0).

19.045 Identify the organic cause of Section 19 symptoms

A range of organic conditions (for example, cerebral tumors, temporal lobe epilepsy, Huntington's disease and other pathologies) can be associated with Section 19 symptoms. These can be indicated for individual items by using the optional attributional scale. For the section as a whole, the letter identifying the ICD - 10 chapter, and up to three digits, should be entered at item **19.045, 20.077, 20.079** or **20.081**. A list of ICD - 10 categories is provided in the Appendix.

Psychoactive substances rated in Sections 11 and 12, such as alcohol, cocaine, and amphetamines, which can be associated with the symptoms should also be rated in Sections 11 or 12, but can also be indicated for individual items with the etiology attribution option.

Dementias and delirium and other cognitive disorders are rated in Section 21.

20 Further information for classification of Part Two disorders

20.001 - 20.013   Course items

Detailed instructions are given in the SCAN manual. These ratings are extremely important for classification using ICD-10 and DSM-IV systems.

20.014 - 20.044   Checklists for Acute and Induced Psychosis, Schizotypal Disorder, and Simple Schizophrenia

20.045 - 20.060   Attributions of cause for Sections 16-19 symptoms during the period

Both ICD-10 and DSM-III, III-R and IV, require the exclusion of attributions of "cause", particularly in relation to the judged effects of psychoactive substances and alcohol, other treatments, physical (or "organic") disease, and psychosocial stressors and adversity. Users of SCAN who wish to make use of such classification systems must therefore attempt to consider the grounds for making judgements of this kind, here in relation to Part Two symptoms. Although opportunity to do so is available at the item level using the etiology scale and optional ratings boxes in earlier sections, and at section level at the end of each section, Section 20 allows the user to re-rate these at a syndromal level, in relation to each Section of SCAN, for the purposes of classification. As far as is practicable, such attributional ratings should be delayed until the "causal" status of any attribution can be established with reasonable certainty. See text of Manual for rules for rating attributions, nature of attribution and quality of data available.

Also see note on the rating of organic and other attributions of cause at items **13.033 - 13.048** (page 120) in this Glossary. The same rules should be applied to Part Two item ratings.

20.061 - 20.066   Identify organic causes and rerate interference

The severity, time relationship and degree of interference caused by symptoms and syndromes can be recorded in SCAN within individual Sections. Here the examiner may exercise clinical judgement, taking account of all the information available at the examination, to reconsider which section appears to be the most clinically significant in Part Two. If necessary re - check ratings of relationships between syndromes within individual Sections (**17.014** and **19.036**).

20.067 - 20.075   Psychosocial attributions influencing the overall manifestation of symptoms throughout Sections 16 to 26

As in Part One, psychosocial attributions that are thought to have effected the manifestation of symptoms throughout SCAN Part Two can be rated here. Specific ratings of stress induced psychosis should also be considered at items **20.018, 20.026 - 20.028**.

20.076 - 20.091   Negative Syndrome and Items

The clinical concept addressed by this subsection is that of a putative subtype of schizophrenia characterized by primary and persistent negative symptoms ("the deficit syndrome"). Rating of the negative syndrome is optional and is included for research purposes. There is overlap with some items in Sections 22-24 and other items but the ratings for the negative syndrome are intended to be based not only on the presence of the negative symptom but must also include a clinical judgement as to whether the symptom is primary or secondary, and ascertainment of the duration of the symptom. The symptom must have been present for the preceding 12 months and to have been always present during periods of clinical stability (including chronic psychotic states). The symptom may or may not have been detectable during transient episodes of acute psychotic disorganization or decompensation.

Symptom items have similar rating points with specific criteria. Etiologic attribution for each negative symptom item is rated in the following item with a 6 - point rating scale which allows atribution of more than one factor. This is different from the general etiology scale used for optional rating of attribution for other SCAN items. The attribution scale is:

Attribution Scale for Negative Syndrome

0   Primary symptom, not secondary to other factors
1   Due to anxiety
2   Due to drug effects
4   Due to suspiciousness (and other psychotic symptoms)
8   Due to mental retardation
16 Due to depression

To score more than one of these just circle the items and add up the numbers for a total score to be recorded. This number can always be uniquely decomposed into the original constituents.

20.076   Restricted affect

This item is to be rated on the basis of what is observed in the interview and by others who have longterm contact with the subject. Restricted affect refers to observed behaviors rather than the subject's subjective experience. Specifically, one rates:

-   A relatively expressionless face, or unchanging facial expression

- Reduced expressive gestures when emotional material is discussed
- Diminished vocal inflection

It is important to distinguish primary restricted affect from a guarded speaking style which is caused by suspiciousness, or a relatively normally reticence or shyness in an interview. These secondary features should be distinguished from a truly restricted affect, and should lead to a rating of 0 or 1 on this item. Information from other sources may be helpful in making such distinctions.

20.077 Restricted affect - attribution

20.078 Diminished emotional range

Under this item, one rates the intensity and range of a subject's (subjective) emotional experience. This item should be distinguished from the capacity to display affect, which is rated under restricted affect rather than here. An inability to experience pleasure of dysphoria of any kind are rated. For instance, a subject who seems to experience little pleasure because of feeling tortured by auditory hallucinations would not be considered to have a diminished emotional range.

It is important to distinguish a primary diminution of emotional range from a normal reticence with strangers, including professionals.

20.079 Diminished emotional range - attribution

20.080 Poverty of speech

Poverty of speech is rated on the basis of behavior during the interview. The deliberate withholding of speech, for instance on the basis of persecutory beliefs or a relatively normal reticence with strangers, would not be considered primary poverty of speech. The rating is based both on the number of words used and the amount of information conveyed, including that information which is volunteered and is not absolutely required by a literal answer to a question. The abnormality sometimes called poverty of content of speech is not rated here. Poverty of content of speech is used to mean an adequate amount of speech or number of words with little information conveyed because of vagueness or repetitive, stereotyped, or cliche-ridden speech.

20.081 Poverty of speech - attribution

20.082 Curbing of interests

This item is used to rate the degree to which the subject is interested in the world around him or her, both ideas and events. The rating should be based on both the subject's behavior and thoughts. Being interested in the world around one is different from having a good fund of knowledge.

The subject may display a diminished range if interests or a diminished depth of interests; either impairment may be considered pathological. However, a great depth of interest in a narrow range of topics (such as found among researchers!) will usually not be considered pathological. A pathological preoccupation with psychotic goals may limit curiosity or interest in other things, but this is not curbing of interests as intended here, as the subject is clearly still lively with regard to this area of function. The subject with an intense but apparently pathological interest in an unrealistic goal, which guides both thought and action, does not display curbing of interests.

20.083 Curbing of interests - attribution

20.084 Diminished sense of purpose

Under this item one is attempting to rate: 1) the degree to which the subject posits goals for his/her life; 2) the extent to which the subject fails to initiate or sustain goal - directed activity due to inadequate drive; and 3) the amount of time passed in aimless inactivity. Whether or not the goal is realistic is irrelevant. However, the subject with a superficial commitment to a goal - i.e., who only pays lip service to a socially acceptable goal - should be considered to have a diminished sense of purpose. It may be important to distinguish between activity for which the subject provides the impetus, and one for which another person (such as a family member) provides it.

In many instances, it is crucial, although difficult, to distinguish a diminished sense of purpose from a subject's 1) psychotic disorganization or 2) feeling overwhelmed from what would, for most people, be a relatively small amount of effort. If a subject has an impaired sense of purpose (a negative symptom), but this is considered secondary to psychosis, he or she would receive a 2 or 3 here, and a "4 - Due to suspiciousness (and other psychotic symptoms) " under item 10, "Diminished sense of purpose - primary or secondary."

20.085 Diminished sense of purpose - attribution

20.086 Diminished social drive

This item is used to rate the degree to which the person seeks or wishes for social interaction. The avoidant subject, who longs for social contact and fitfully seeks it but is made uncomfortable by it, is not considered to have diminished social drive. The rating should consider the subject's internal experience, statements, and behaviors. Social success is not rated here. Many schizophrenics have serious social disabilities, but most socially impaired person, schizophrenic or otherwise, usually continue to seek social interaction of some kind. The term does not refer to social withdrawal that is present only during psychotic episodes, or withdrawal that is due to suspiciousness, an effort to decrease stimuli, or any other factor other than a lack of interest in relationships.

20.087 Diminished social drive - attribution

20.088 Poor social performance

This item is distinguished from diminished social drive although it may be related. It assesses actual social performance rather than the effort or interest to interact socially.

20.089 Poor nonverbal communication

This item differs from poverty of speech in assessing the non - verbal components of communication. For example, gestures, voice modulation, timing, facial expression, etc.

20.090 Poor self care

This item is self-explanatory.

20.091 Psychomotor slowing

This item as well as the previous items is necessary for the ICD-10 diagnosis of Residual Schizophrenia. It assesses decreased motor activity associated with slowed mentation. Slowed mentation must be inferred from responsiveness to verbal and other cognitive interactions with the environment (or perhaps functional brain imaging).

20.092 Adequacy of ratings in sections 16 - 20

See rules for making this rating at the end of Section 13, page 120.

21 Cognitive impairment and decline

GENERAL POINTS ABOUT SECTION 21

Section 21 deals chiefly with cognitive impairments and decline. These occur in neurotic, affective and psychotic disorders as well as in disorders with a more overt 'organic' basis.

At this point of the interview it will usually be apparent whether there is evidence of cognitive problems. Clinical observation together with answers to questions in Sections 0 (socio-demographic), 1 (introduction) and throughout Part One of SCAN should be sufficient to allow a clinical judgement. Such evidence will be one of several reasons to continue below the cut-off.

Since most of the severe cognitive problems will be associated with disorders in sub-chapter F0 of ICD-10, it is important to be aware of the definition of the term 'organic' given there, which is repeated in the introduction to this Glossary. The use of the term does not imply that conditions in other sub-chapters are 'non-organic' in the sense of not having a cerebral substrate. It "means no more and no less than that the syndrome so classified can be attributed to an independently diagnosable cerebral or systemic disease. The term 'symptomatic' refers to those organic mental disorders in which cerebral involvement is secondary to a systemic, extracerebral disease." Thus two codes are needed; one for the syndrome and one for the postulated causal disease, trauma or other insult to the brain.

In PSE10, only causes or pathologies thought to be responsible for dementia, delirium or amnesic syndromes are entered in Section 21 itself. Acute intoxication or acute poisoning causing symptoms of cognitive impairment or disorder, due to substances other than those rated in Sections 11 and 12, should be rated at items **21.118** and **21.123**.

Attributions of an organic cause for somatoform, dissociative, neurotic, affective and psychotic symptom types are made in Sections 13 and 20. A qualification to this is made only for symptom types that are rated as caused by alcohol (Section 11) or by the drugs listed in Section 12. For example, if symptoms of anxiety are thought to be due to amphetamine, the relevant symptom items would be rated present or uncertain as instructed in the Glossary, the attribution of an organic cause would be made at item **13.033 - 13.048** and the substance identified at item **12.034.5**. However, if the anxiety symptoms are thought to be due to thyrotoxicosis, the ICD-10 code would be entered at item **13.049, 13.051, 13.053**. The same principle holds for alcohol or drug-induced hallucinosis.

Note that anxiety or depression thought to be precipitated by a psychological mechanism, for example, awareness of failing cognitive powers, would not be grounds for an attribution of 'organic anxiety' or 'organic depression'.

Finally, it should be emphasized that the cut-off point should be passed whenever there is any possibility that cognitive problems are present and that the items in Section 21 must be rated independently of the interviewer's own preliminary diagnostic formulations. If for any reason the screening process does not include the full Mini-Mental State Examination, the reasons for this must be clearly recorded at **21.001**.

CUT-OFF POINT

21.001 Evidence of cognitive decline or impairment

Carefully follow the instructions in the Manual on how to proceed. Rate (0) if examiner has decided not to proceed with specific cognitive screening. It is preferred that the reasons for doing so are recorded.

21.002 Verbal trails test

This is a test for possible 'subcortical' dementia, that may not be picked up in the Mini-Mental State Examination. Full instructions are provided in the Manual.

MINI-MENTAL STATE EXAMINATION

Before starting the Mini-Mental State Examination it may be helpful to point out to R that some of the standard questions have to be very simple. They are included so as to assess all levels of memory and carry no particular implication.

The score for correct answers for items included in the MMS is shown on the right hand side of the rating boxes. Items **21.014**, **21.023**, and **21.025** are not included in the MMS total. Item **21.027** is provided for hand scoring of the MMS total, which is required in order to decide on whether or not to CUT to Section 22. The computer program will also provide the sum for subsequent analysis.

21.003 - 21.007 Orientation in time

Start by asking R the date. Rate correct answers as (1) and incorrect as (0). If R is unable to answer because of cognitive impairment rate (0) unless due to disorders affecting speech, movement or motivation (e.g. Parkinson's syndrome); then rate (8).

Orientation in place

21.008 Ask R to name the county or region or district where the interview takes place.

21.009 R should also name the town, village or city.

21.010 The name of the street where the interview takes place, or some local landmark if there is no street name.

21.011 The name of the building (hospital, surgery, house, block of apartments, etc.) where the interview takes place.

21.012 The name of the country.

Rate correct answers (1) and incorrect (0). If R is unable to answer because of cognitive impairment rate (0), if due to disorders affecting speech, movement or motivation, rate (8). If there are special circumstances (e.g. recent admission to hospital) explaining why R cannot answer items **21.010 - 21.012**, rate (7).

21.013 Name three objects

Be sure that the respondent is attentive. Read the question slowly. Do not repeat the objects until after the first trial. Repeating the objects in a different order is acceptable. Scoring in **21.013** (maximum 3) is based solely on the first trial. If R does not repeat the items on the first attempt, ask for another try.

21.014 Number of trials (registration)

Enter the number of extra trials. The purpose of making up to five trials is to allow short-term memory to be assessed later.

21.015 Serial sevens

This and the following item are focused on the respondent's attention and concentration. However, defects in short-term memory, disturbed spatial ability and primary acalculia (loss of the ability to appreciate or manipulate numbers as symbols), as well as dysphasias may influence rating of this item. The interviewer should read the question slowly, and he should repeat it if the respondent does not understand. Rate (1) for each correct and (0) for each incorrect answer (maximum score=5). If a subtraction is wrong but the previous and subsequent responses are correct, this counts as only one error e.g. 93, 88, 81, 74, 67 (score=4). If there are two mistakes e.g. 96, 88, 81, 74, 67 this counts as two errors (score=3). If the respondent is aware that he has made an error and corrects it, accept this correction. Similarly, if he gets an answer right and then changes his mind, count it as an error. If the subject is not able to co-operate because of a disorder of speech, movement or motivation, rate (6). If R is unable to co-operate due to cognitive impairment, rate (0). In subjects who cannot attempt for educational reasons (illiteracy), rate (7).

21.016 Spell 'world' backwards

Read the question slowly. Say the whole word at first and then spell it for the respondent. Repeat the spelling if the respondent asks. Rate the number of correct letters in the right place (maximum score 5). Transposition of two letters counts as two errors. Each extra or omitted letter counts as an error.

21.017   Recall 3 objects

Ask the respondent to name the three objects (**21.013**). Maximum score 3. R must not be helped in any way, but should be reassured if there are mistakes. Changing the order of items does not count as an error.

21.018 - 21.025   LANGUAGE COMPREHENSION

The purpose of these items is to make a general assessment of problems in understanding spoken and written language, and in the expression of speech. These problems occur predominantly in people suffering from organic mental disorders. However, some patients with 'functional' psychiatric disorders may also have difficulty in accomplishing these simple tasks.

21.018   Name 'pencil'

21.019   Name 'watch'

R may be completely unable to name these simple objects (**21.018** and **21.019**). This may be due to nominal dysphasia (amnesic aphasia). R may also attempt to name these objects but use a different word or make up a word (neologism), or mispronounce the word, or substitute syllables (paraphasia). These problems may indicate primary motor dysphasia (Broca) or primary sensory dysphasia (Wernicke). Rating can also be affected by visual object agnosia, i.e. the inability to recognize an object by sight.

Rate incorrect answers as (0) and correct as (1). If R is unable to attempt to answer because of cognitive impairment rate (0). If there are difficulties in naming these objects explained by motor or motivational disorders, rate (6). If R is unable to attempt because of disorders of sight, rate (8).

21.020   Repeat 'No ifs, ands, or buts'

This item concerns the repetition of spoken language. Mistakes similar to those mentioned in **21.023 - 21.024** may occur. Primary motor or sensory dysphasia, subcortical motor dysphasia and conduction dysphasia are the main causes of errors. The interviewer must enunciate clearly, including the "s" at the end of ifs, ands and buts. Any omitted "s" or any other error counts. Rate errors as (0) and correct answer as (1). If the subject is unable to attempt to answer because of cognitive impairment rate (0). If there are difficulties in performing this task explained by motor or motivational disorders, rate (6).

21.021   Fold paper in half, etc.

R is presented with a blank sheet of paper. The full statement is read aloud before handing it over. The interviewer should not repeat the instructions or coach. The paper should be directly in front of the respondent, so that R reaches out to take it. The interviewer observes which hand is used and whether the other two instructions are followed. The item concerns both understanding of spoken language and praxis. If there are any mistakes or omissions in carrying out the tasks, this might indicate pure-word deafness (subcortical auditory dysphasia), or apraxia (ideational or ideomotor apraxia).

Code the number of tasks that the subject carried out correctly. If R is unable to attempt because of cognitive impairment rate (0). If difficulties in performing the tasks are explained by motor or motivational disorders, rate (6). If R is unable or has difficulties in performing the tasks because of disorders of hearing, rate (8).

21.022 Read sentence, 'Close your eyes'

For a rating of (1) it does not matter whether or not the respondent reads the sentence out loud. The response is correct if R follows the instructions correctly. If R does not read or follow the order, rate (0). Afterwards, the interviewer may need to tell the respondent to open his or her eyes.

The item assesses the understanding of written language. An error in this item may indicate the presence of pure word blindness (alexia) or primary sensory dysphasia (Wernicke). If R is unable to attempt because of cognitive impairment rate (0). If there are difficulties in reading and performing the task explained by motor or motivational disorders, rate (6). If the subject cannot read because of educational problems rate (7), if problems with sight, rate (8).

21.023 Repeat 21.022

Follow instructions in the Manual.

21.024 Write, then read, a sentence

21.025 Ever able to write properly

These items test writing ability. Difficulties with the test may indicate "agraphia" i.e. the inability to write. R is asked to write a sentence without being helped in any way. Rate (0) if the result is completely unsuccessful, and (1) if important elements of the sentence (e.g. subject or verb) are missing. If R is unable to attempt because of cognitive impairment rate (0). If there are difficulties in performing the task explained by motor or motivational disorders, rate (6). Rate educational factors that might influence the result here.

21.026 Copy pentagrams

The interviewer should produce a piece of paper with the pentagram figures and hand it to the respondent for copying. The copy is correct if it shows two 5-sided figures with corners pointing outwards and an overlap between with four sides. The following elements are involved in carrying out this task:

(a) understanding written language;

(b) praxis;
(c) construction.

Defects in any of these may affect the result. Rate (0) if the result does not correspond to the instructions above and (1) if it does. If the subject is unable to attempt because of cognitive impairment rate (0). If there are difficulties in performing the task explained by motor or motivational disorders, rate (6). If R cannot perform the task because of visual problems, rate (8).

21.027 Sum scores in marked boxes

21.028 Underestimation of cognitive abilities

These items are self-explanatory.

MEMORY

21.029 Repeat naming of three objects after 5 minutes

21.030 Subjectively described memory problems

Make a general rating of memory problems in this item. Rate only the patient's experience. However, if it is indicated, use evidence available from other sources to cross-examine the patient. Mild memory problems arising mainly from inattention, worry, anxiety, etc., are rated (1). Rate severe and persisting memory problems as (2). Note that the severity of memory problems does not depend on the cause. Memory problems can be severe in disorders other than those listed in F0 of ICD-10 (e.g. depressive pseudodementia). If R denies memory problems but these are found present on testing (i.e. MMS) rate (3). If R is unable to answer because of cognitive impairment, rate (4). Rate (7) if the memory problem (which would usually be mild) has had no 'onset', e.g. if R has always been 'absent-minded'.

21.031 Adoption of methods to compensate for memory deficits

Rate the strategies R adopts in order to overcome memory problems, e.g. using notebooks and lists, adopting strict routines so as not to forget even simple tasks that would normally be undertaken without conscious effort, etc. Rate the extent to which R is unable to carry on an everyday routine without such aids, irrespective of how successful the strategies are. Rate 0, 1 and 2 as in **21.031**. If unable to answer because of cognitive impairment rate 3.

21.032 Forgetting names of intimates

This is a more serious type of forgetting. Mild, transient forgetting, usually due to worry, anxiety or inattention, is rated (1). Rate (2) if R is unable to remember the names of children, spouse, parents, close friends, but R is aware of. Rate (3) if the subject is unable to answer the question because of cognitive impairment. Use all available information to rate this symptom.

21.033 Disorientation near home

R is unable to find his way back home if left alone near home. Local landmarks are no longer familiar. If R does make mistakes but manages, for example to get to the shops and back without help, rate (1). Rate (2) if R has had to have help to get home and is at risk when out. If R does not go out or is not allowed out because of severe cognitive impairment, or is always accompanied, rate (3).

21.034 More serious forgetting

A few instances of behavior that might become problematic, if repeated in more hazardous circumstances, could be rated (1). If memory lapses due to cognitive impairment are clearly hazardous, e.g. food is left in the oven to burn, the gas or the electric fire are left on in potentially dangerous circumstances, etc., rate (2). Rate (3) if the patient is not able to answer the question because of cognitive impairment, or is always supervised to prevent dangerous consequences.

21.035 Repeat numbers

This item assesses 'immediate memory', the reproduction of material that falls within the span of attention. This can be affected by disorders of memory, concentration, attention, anxiety, depression, etc. Code the number of correct digits irrespective of the order. If the subject is unable to attempt because of cognitive impairment rate (0). If there are difficulties in performing the task explained by motor or motivational disorders, rate (6). If the subject cannot hear, rate (8).

21.036 Name present Prime Minister (President)

This item assesses recent memory, spanning longer time periods than **21.029**. Rate (0) for correct and (1) for incorrect answers. If the subject is unable to attempt because of cognitive impairment rate (0). If there are difficulties in performing the task explained by motor or motivational disorders, rate (6).

REMOTE MEMORY

21.037 R's date of birth

Other tests of remote memory.

Local equivalents that test widely known historical knowledge, and are of increasing difficulty, may be devised and used for testing. Up to 12 additional items may be added. No algorithms are available. Rate also remote memory at **21.095**.

LANGUAGE USE

21.038 Read: 'People in glass houses'

21.039   Ever able to read a sentence

These items refer as in **21.025** to language use. Word-blindness (alexia), dysphasia (either motor or sensory dysphasia) may account for the inability or difficulty of the respondent to read the sentence. R is either unable to read the sentence at all (rate 0), or reads correctly only a few words but not the whole sentence (rate 1). If the whole sentence is read correctly, rate (2). If the subject is unable to attempt because of cognitive impairment rate (9). If there are difficulties in reading explained by motor or motivational disorders, rate (6). Rate educational factors which may influence the results here.

21.040   Name as many animals as possible

Verbal fluency is assessed in this item. Respondents with dysphasia, perseveration, memory problems, disorders of volition, attention, concentration, and serious depression, may have considerable difficulties in completing this test. Record the number of different animals named in 60 seconds. If R is unable to attempt because of cognitive impairment rate (00). If there are difficulties in performing the task due to motor or motivational disorders, rate (66).

21.041   Name three pictures

The respondent should recognize the three objects (spectacles, shoe, suitcase). The notes for items **21.018** and **21.019** apply here as well. Record the number of items correctly identified (1-3). If the subject is unable to attempt because of cognitive impairment rate (0). If there are difficulties in performing the task explained by motor or motivational disorders, rate (6). If the subject cannot attempt because of problems with sight, rate (8).

21.042   Write then read sentence

21.043   Ever able to write properly

21.044   Simple addition

21.045   Ever able to do simple addition

21.046   Simple subtraction

21.047   Ever able to do simple subtraction

The respondent is asked to do simple arithmetic like addition (**21.044**) and subtraction (**21.046**). As for **21.015**, difficulty can be due to disordered attention and concentration, problems with memory, disturbed spatial ability and acalculia. Rate correct answers as (1) and incorrect as (0). If the subject is unable to attempt because of cognitive impairment rate (0). If there are difficulties in performing the task explained by motor or motivational disorders, rate (6). Rate educational factors that might influence the results at **21.045** and **21.047**.

PRAXIS

Rate (0) on the items if the test was not performed correctly. In **21.048** rate (1) for correct completion of the task. In **21.050** a rating of (1) indicates that only one of the two actions was performed correctly. If the tasks are carried out correctly rate each (2). If R is unable to attempt because of cognitive impairment rate (0). If there are difficulties in performing the tasks explained by motor or motivational disorders, rate (6). If R cannot hear and therefore cannot attempt, rate (8).

21.048 Nod head

21.049 Wave 'good-bye'

21.050 Touch right ear with left hand

Like **21.021**, these items involve both comprehension of spoken language and praxis. Problems in carrying out the tasks may therefore indicate difficulties or inability in understanding spoken language (pure word deafness) or disorder in the execution of voluntary acts (apraxia). Errors in **21.048** indicate the presence of ideomotor apraxia (inability to organize voluntary movement in space and time) while in **21.050** ideational apraxia is also present (inability to carry out coordinated sequences of actions).

21.051 Hand praxis

Follow instructions in manual. Take account of any physical abnormality that could limit R's ability to carry out the task.

ABSTRACTION

21.052 Similarity between an apple and a banana

21.053 Similarity between a boat and a car

Abstract thinking is assessed by these items. This can be affected in organic and 'functional' mental disorders. Rate correct answers (2) and incorrect (0). Rate partially correct (1), for example apple and banana are both yellow or both have skin. If the subject is unable to attempt because of cognitive impairment rate (0). If there are difficulties in performing the task explained by motor or motivational disorders, rate (6).

21.054 'People in glass houses'

Instructions are at **21.057**.

21.055 'A rolling stone gathers no moss'

See **21.057**.

21.056   'Many hands make light work'

See **21.057**.

21.057   Bizarre answers to proverbs

Like item **21.058**, the interpretation of proverbs known to nearly everybody helps the examiner to assess difficulties in abstract thinking. Dysphasic disorders also affect the answers to these questions either due to difficulties of understanding spoken language, or because of difficulties in the production of speech by the respondent. A rating of (0) means that the respondent gives a concrete literal interpretation without understanding the abstract meaning.

Rate (1) if the respondent gives an abstract interpretation indicating that the respondent has some understanding of the abstract nature of the task but gets the meaning wrong (e.g. in **21.054**: '*People are fragile, like glass*'). Rate appropriate answers ('*Don't accuse others if you have faults yourself*') as (2). If R is unable to attempt because of cognitive impairment rate (0). If there are difficulties in interpreting the proverb explained by motor or motivational disorders, rate (6).

Rate item **21.057** if the answer to the proverbs is bizarre or absurd or delusional. Rate (3) if all answers are bizarre, (2) if much bizarre content occurs, (1) if answer made is somewhat clear, and (0) if all answers are clear.

FUND OF KNOWLEDGE

Some of the following items are intended to be difficult and therefore are designed to test level of education and indirectly intelligence.

21.058   How tall is the average man

Answers to this item can be wildly wrong if respondents have severe cognitive disorder, especially severe amnesia and acalculia. Mental retardation, disorders in the autistic spectrum (particularly Asperger syndrome), and psychotic conditions may also lead to strange answers.

Rate correct answers (2). Answers that deviate somewhat from expected correct answers are rated (1). Wildly wrong answers (e.g. 10 meters) are rated (0). If the subject is unable to attempt the task because of cognitive impairment rate (9). If there are difficulties in performing the task explained by motor or motivational disorders, rate (6). If educational problems account for errors, rate (8).

21.059   Color of a clear sky

21.060   Capital of Italy

21.061 Function of lungs

21.062 Function of barometer/ thermometer

It may be necessary to use a local equivalent, but if so, it should not be an easy subject.

FRONTO / SUBCORTICAL TESTS

21.063 Hand sequencing test

Follow instructions in manual, taking account of any physical impairment.

21.064 Finger tapping trial test

Follow instructions in manual, taking account of any physical impairment.

LEVEL OF CONSCIOUSNESS

21.065 Level of consciousness

Rate disturbances of consciousness independently of type. Rate states of impaired consciousness (e.g. clouding) and altered consciousness (e.g. twilight states). Rate (1) if the disturbance is moderate or severe but transient and (2) for severe persistent disturbance.

21.066 Drowsiness

The state of the respondent is one of apathy, with few spontaneous movements, apart from defensive or avoiding movements when painful stimuli are applied, or movements correcting posture. R does not speak spontaneously, and responds verbally to voices or stimuli with dysarthric speech or mumbling. R is moderately disoriented. Although R falls asleep if left alone, arousal is easy when spoken to loudly, or by physical contact. Reflexes are maintained, but muscular tone, swallowing and often coughing reflexes are reduced. Rate (1) if the disturbance is moderate or severe but transient and (2) for severe persistent disturbance.

21.067 Clouding or daze

This is the mildest stage of impairment of consciousness. R is sleepy and thinking, attention, perception and memory are affected. Nevertheless, R can obey simple instructions and move about and, to some extent act appropriately. When sleeping, R can easily be aroused by voice or physical contact, but is disoriented when woken. There is little spontaneous speech. Rate (1) if the disturbance is moderate or severe but transient and (2) for severe persistent disturbance.

21.068 Akinetic mutism

Akinetic mutism ('coma vigil') is seen in people with lesions (usually tumors) in the diencephalon and the upper brain stem. The symptom resembles stupor seen in psychiatric disorders. The patient lies immobile and mute but the eyes are vigilant, observing the examiner steadily or following moving objects. The patient is mute or answers only by whispering or monosyllables. There are no voluntary movements although the patient can make unsuccessful attempts to follow simple commands. This state is often followed by coma. Rate (1) if the disturbance is moderate or severe but transient and (2) for severe persistent disturbance. Rate dissociative stupor at item **2.056**. Other stupor not associated with cognitive disorder is rated at item **22.006**.

21.069 Coma

This is the most severe disturbance in the continuum of impaired consciousness. The patient's eyes are closed and he or she cannot be aroused. There is no response to external stimuli and no spontaneous movements. Muscular tone is diminished and reflexes are progressively lost as coma becomes deeper. Rate in this item both coma and semi-coma (partial, incomplete, non- purposive response to stimulation, with light and corneal reflexes still present). Distinguish from deep sleep, in the sense that in the latter the patient can be woken and there is still mental activity in the form of dreams which leave some memory trace, and stupor. In coma, the eyes remain shut even after strong stimuli, do not resist passive opening, and do not appear to be watchful or follow moving objects, while movements, if they exist, are not purposeful, and there is no subsequent recall of events as in stupor. Rate (1) if the disturbance is moderate or severe but transient and (2) for severe persistent disturbance.

21.070 Illusions when clouded

In delirium, clouded consciousness is usually accompanied by disordered perception usually in the form of visual illusions and hallucinations. Illusions and misinterpretations in the visual field may take the form of macropsia, micropsia, or distortions of shape and position of objects or even the patient's own body. Visual hallucinations may be simple (flashes of light, geometrical patterns, colors), or fully, formed hallucinations of scenes, animals or people. In delirium tremens the patient often sees small animals (rats, snakes, etc.) or insects which appear in colorful and vivid forms. R may also see threatening or amusing scenes from the past. These disturbances of perception are fleeting and transient but they are accepted fully by the patient who often reacts emotionally to them. Rate (1) if the disturbance is moderate or severe but transient and (2) for severe persistent disturbance. Rate attribution of delirium tremens in 11.29.

21.071 Fantastic ideas when clouded

Thought processes are characteristically affected in clouded consciousness. In the early stages slowing of thought and difficulty in formulating complex ideas are the main problems. Later on, logic and reasoning become impaired and thinking becomes concrete and literal. Thought becomes impoverished and stereotyped and organization of thought is weakened, resulting in fragmentation of thought and finally incoherence. As logic weakens, the patient's sense of reality is affected in the sense that there is no distinction between inner and outer worlds, or between thoughts and perceptions. R cannot attach any significance and understanding to the immediate situation or to events happening outside. Subjective experiences, ideas and false perceptions dominate the content of consciousness. R expresses bizarre ideas and fantasies and interprets external cues falsely. Eventually, poorly elaborated delusions of reference or persecution appear and dominate the content of thought. They tend to be transient but in rare instances continue to be held with conviction even after the state of disturbed consciousness subsides.

Rate (1) if the disturbance is moderate or severe but transient and (2) for severe persistent disturbance. Rate attribution of delirium tremens in **11.031**.

21.072 Psychomotor disturbance when clouded

In most cases of clouded consciousness there is diminished motor behavior with apathy and little spontaneous activity. Actions are carried out in an automatic manner. There is diminished or absent response to external cues and speech is slow, sparse, slurred, and often incoherent, with perseveration and signs of dysphasia. This picture often alternates with the opposite, a picture of excessive reaction which is often triggered by subjective events such as hallucinations or delusional ideas. There is hyperactivity, restlessness, and noisy behavior, with excessive startle reactions. R may engage in repetitive purposeless behavior (e.g. picking movements), or imaginary conversation arising from hallucinatory experiences, or reacting to delusional ideas, e.g. trying to hide or escape from imaginary enemies. There is often excitement, shouting, laughing or crying, pressure of speech, incoherence and flight of ideas. States of apathy and hyperactivity may change rapidly into one another.

Rate (1) if the disturbance is recent and mild or transient; (2) for marked disturbance. Rate attribution of delirium tremens at **11.031**.

21.073 Reversed sleep-wake cycle

This disturbance is typical in patients in states of clouded consciousness. Symptoms, especially when they are mild, worsen at night, with fatigue and decreased environmental stimulation. When the examiner visits the patient at daytime, there is a milder picture than described by relatives or night nurses. The patient often suffers from insomnia or total loss of nocturnal sleep with sleepiness during the daytime. There are often vivid nightmares which are experienced as continuing in the form of hallucinations after waking.

Rate (1) if the disturbance is moderate or severe but transient and (2) for severe persistent disturbance.

21.074 Acute intoxication on examination

Toxic effects of alcohol and drugs covered in Section 12 are rated at items **11.028 - 11.031** and **12.043**. Other intoxication or poisoning affecting cognitive functions is rated here. Accidental drinking of surgical spirit by a patient with severe dementia, would for example be rated here. Take into account slurred speech, nystagmus, flushed face, incoordination, alteration of behavior (agitation or hyperactivity or apathy and introverted behavior) depending on the type of drug taken.

Rate (1) if the disturbance is moderate and (2) for severe disturbance. Enter the diagnosis (ICD-10) of the toxic agent at item **21.075**.

21.075 Identify cause of symptoms rated at 21.074

Enter ICD-10 code for agent. Do not include if due to alcohol or substance rated in Section 11 or 12.

21.076 Fugue

Rate here fugues other than those of a dissociative nature which are rated at item **2.055**. The fugues rated here occur usually in patients suffering from organic mental states, e.g. epilepsy. Respondents with dissociative fugue are usually well preserved in comparison to those with epileptic fugues, who are often found dirty, dishevelled and neglected. Those with dissociative fugues tend to travel to places with some emotional significance instead of aimlessly wandering. Use all available information from informants and case-records to make the rating. Rate (1) if the disturbance has occurred.

OVERALL RATINGS OF COGNITIVE IMPAIRMENT O.E.

The following ratings are been made on the basis of the information the interviewer has collected during interview, especially Section 21.

21.077 Memory impairment overall O.E.

Take into account especially ratings at **21.003 - 21.013, 21.029 - 21.037,** and **21.017**. Rate all forms of memory impairment, irrespective of the kind of amnesia (global, retrograde, anterograde) and the type of memory affected (immediate, recent or remote memory).

Rate (1) if the patient's disorder is moderate but the loss of memory has left areas of activity and time periods relatively intact. A rating of (2) means a severe disturbance of memory covering even remote time periods and seriously affecting the life of the respondent to the extent that assistance or supervision are required.

21.078 Loss of intellectual functions overall O.E.

Use all available information from the interview or case records as well as accounts by informants. Take into account:

(a) loss of the ability to understand the environment;
(b) loss of the ability to understand and complete linguistic and arithmetic tasks;

(c) diminished attention and concentration;
(d) diminished drive, self-expression and spontaneity;
(e) decrease in interests and activities resulting in diminished social interaction and social withdrawal;
(f) decreased ability to produce ideas using past and present experiences;
(g) decreased ability to distinguish past from present;
(h) impaired logic, judgement, capacity for abstraction and perspicuity.

Rate (1) if the patient's disorder is moderate but the loss of intellectual function has left areas of activity relatively intact. A rating of (2) means a severe disturbance of intellect affecting seriously the life of the respondent so that assistance or supervision are required.

21.079 Disorientation overall (time, place, person)

Use all available information from interview (e.g. answers to demographic items in Section 0, items **21.003 - 21.013**) as well as information from case-records and informants.

Rate (1) if the patient is moderately disoriented or is severely disoriented but not in all areas. A rating of (2) means a severe disorientation in all three areas affecting seriously the life of the respondent so that assistance or supervision are required. In the most severe cases the patient loses even a sense of personal identity.

21.080 Perseveration

Perseverative errors occur usually in patients with primary sensory dysphasia (Wernicke), but can occur in other disorders as well. Rate independently of possible origin. R's speech is interspersed with words or phrases used in earlier times that cannot be discarded, or there are useless repetitions of words.

Rate (1) if there are few errors; (2) if frequent.

21.081 Retrograde amnesia

Memory for past experiences, covering time periods from a few seconds, minutes or hours (e.g. in the case of head injury) to months or years before the onset of the impairment (e.g. in the case of organic amnesic syndrome). These are called short and long retrograde amnesia respectively. Retrograde amnesia is usually dense, but it also may be incomplete and patchy.

Rate (1) if the disturbance is moderate, or severe but transient, and (2) for severe persistent disturbance.

21.082 Confabulation

Confabulations are false memories. They occur in clear consciousness, usually in patients with amnesia. Respondents give a coherent but entirely false account of some recent event or experience. Confabulations may be true memories misplaced in time or context, intended to fill memory gaps. However, they may possess a fantastic quality (like those rated separately in **19.019** because not accompanied by amnesia) in which the patient describes events, experiences or adventures which are unlikely to be real.

Rate (1) if the disturbance is of moderate severity; (2) for severe disturbance where large areas of recent memory are covered by confabulation.

21.083 Relatively isolated memory impairment

In this symptom, intellectual functions are intact, as well as level of consciousness and immediate memory (e.g. digit span). The main impairment is in recent memory, with impaired ability to learn new material, and forgetting what is learnt more quickly than normal. New memories cannot be placed into the long-term store. This results in both anterograde and retrograde amnesia of varying density with inability to recall past experiences in reverse order of their occurrence. Memory gaps are often filled by confabulations which are usually misplaced true memories.

Rate (1) if the impairment is of moderate severity; (2) for severe impairment where large areas of recent memory are affected.

21.084 Slowness and difficulty with speech/movement

Include behaviors indicative of retardation of spontaneous and voluntary movement and speech (abulia), up to but not including akinetic mutism or stupor (item **21.068**). Rate only symptoms of organic origin, excluding similar 'functional' disorders (e.g. those rated at items **2.056, 7.005,** and **22.006**). Take into account:

(a) Psychiatric history;
(b) Neurological examination, especially signs of lesions in the diencephalon or upper brain stem;
(c) The presence of any catatonic phenomena;
(d) The level of consciousness;
(e) The presence of depressive or manic affect;
(f) The presence of stress, evidence of motives, and conversion symptoms.

Rate (1) if the disturbance is of moderate severity; R may evidently be trying to overcome an impairment. A rating of 2 is reserved for severe slowing, with only slow brief replies or statements, little voluntary movement, and only simple poorly coordinated responses to commands.

21.085 Slowness and difficulty with thought/comprehension

This symptom accompanies that in item **21.084**. Include only symptoms of organic origin. The patient's thought processes are slowed down as reflected in the viscous and torpid nature of the patient's voice and reactions. Distinguish from similar symptoms accompanying 'functional' disorders. Apply the guidelines for differential definition given at item **21.084**.

Rate (1) if the impairment is of moderate severity; (2) for severe impairment.

21.086   Aphasias, apraxias, etc.

This rating allows a summary rating of the aphasias and apraxias present.

The examiner will by now have acquired most of the information needed to rate the presence of aphasias and apraxias. Consider especially items **21.013 - 21.014, 21.018 - 21.020, 21.022, 21.026, 21.038, 21.040, 21.042** and **21.048**, and take into account other sources such as case-records and informants. Include:

(a) Pure word blindness (alexia without agraphia), i.e. difficulty with understanding what the subject reads;
(b) Pure word dumbness (subcortical motor dysphasia) i.e. difficulty in producing spoken speech with slurring and dysarthria;
(c) Pure agraphia, i.e. inability to write;
(d) Primary sensory dysphasia (Wcrnicke), i.e. impaired comprehension of the spoken language resulting in inability to repeat and respond to commands;
(e) Primary motor dysphasia (Broca), i.e. difficulty or inability to speak;
(f) Nominal dysphasia, i.e. inability to evoke names at will;
(g) Conduction aphasia (syntactical);
(h) Alexia with agraphia, i.e. the inability of both reading and writing;
(i) Jargon aphasia.

For apraxias, consider especially items **21.021, 21.050, 21.049**. Apraxia is the inability to carry out purposive movements or movement complexes in the absence of paresis, lack of coordination, sensory loss, involuntary movements or psychological mechanisms (e.g., psychogenic stupor).

Include:

(a) Ideomotor, i.e. disturbance of voluntary movements as inability of executing although the patient is aware of and can describe the movement that is difficult to perform;
(b) Ideational, i.e. inability to carry out coordinated sequences of actions (e.g. **21.021**).

Rate (1) if the impairment is of moderate severity; (2) for severe impairment associated with aphasias and apraxias.

21.087   Deterioration of self-care on examination

Take into account only the appearance of the patient during interview. Deterioration or loss of self- care becomes evident by malnourishment, inappropriate and inadequate dressing for the time of the year, untidiness, smelling of urine or faeces, deterioration of personal appearance, signs of neglected physical health (including dental care), etc. Rate only behavior related to evident or suspected organic factors. Rate information from case-records or informants at **21.097**.

Rate (1) if the impairment is of moderate severity; (2) for severe impairment.

21.088   Uneven deficits

RECENT CLINICAL HISTORY

21.089 - 21.097   Ratings from case record

These items should be completed on the basis of evidence from case records and informants, and from R if degree of impairment allows.

21.098   Other psychiatric problems associated with dementia

21.099   Relationship of delirium to dementia

PERSONALITY CHANGES

21.100   Personality deterioration

Include only if there have been definite changes from a previous personality, which are clearly associated with cognitive impairment of some kind. Consider decreased emotional control, shallow euphoria, irritability, apathy, disinhibition, suspiciousness, rigidity, neglect of hygiene and changes in sexual behavior. Also consider alteration in the flow and rate of language production. Also include altered sexual behavior like hyposexuality or change in sexual preference. These changes must persist for at least six months.

Rate severity as 1 to 3, according to the degree to which the change is evident to other people and how far elements of the previous personality are preserved.

21.101   Personality changes following encephalitis

Rate present only if personality deterioration (which must be rated 1, 2 or 3 at **21.100**) has followed within 6 months of viral or bacterial encephalitis. There should be residual signs - one or more of the following: paralysis, deafness, aphasia, apraxia, or acalculia.

Since severity is rated at **21.100**, this item is rated either 0 or 1 according to whether the attribution of cause is made; or 8 if the examiner is uncertain.

21.102   Personality changes following head trauma

Rate present only if personality deterioration (which must be rated 1, 2 or 3 at **21.100**) has followed within 4 weeks of head trauma with loss of consciousness. The symptoms will have been rated in Section 2 and 3. There should be three or more of the following items: headache, dizziness, excessive fatigue, noise intolerance, emotional lability, loss of concentration, insomnia and reduced tolerance to alcohol.

Since severity is rated at **21.100**, this item is rated either (0) or (1) according to whether the attribution of cause is made; or (8) if the examiner is uncertain.

21.103 - 21.124   Attribution/s of pathological cause

These items provide an opportunity to enter an attribution of pathology or cause for the symptoms or syndromes specified. A rating of (1) indicates that the examiner has some, but not full, evidence for the attribution; (2) indicates a confident attribution.

MENTAL DISORDERS RATED ELSEWHERE IN PSE10, THAT ARE DUE TO CEREBRAL DISEASE, DAMAGE OR DYSFUNCTION

These disorders include conditions characterized by symptoms rated in Sections of PSE10 other than Section 21. The attribution that there is an 'organic' cause of such symptoms, i.e. that they are caused by a cerebral disorder, either directly, or indirectly via a non-cerebral disorder, is made in Section 13 or 20. (Please read the comment on the use of the term 'organic' in the introduction to this Glossary.)

There is a qualification due to the case of mental disorders caused by the use of alcohol or other substances. The attributions are made in Sections 11 or 12, since that is where substance use is rated and it would be confusing to make the attribution twice. If more detailed attributions are required they can also be made using the etiology scale and option for individual items.

For example, the attribution of an organic cause can be made and the relevant ICD-10 code is specified at item **21.125**. An attribution to amphetamine, however, is made at item appropriate in Section 12 and there should be no need to record anything further.

Similarly, the attribution of organic hallucinosis is made at item **17.034**, but that for alcoholic hallucinosis is made at item **11.019**.

The criteria to be applied when deciding whether there is an organic cause for mental symptoms are set out in Section 13 and 20 of the Glossary, but are summarized here for convenience:

(a)   Evidence of cerebral disorder, damage or dysfunction, whether direct or via non-cerebral disorder.

(b) A temporal relationship between the development or exacerbation of the disease and the onset of the symptoms in the Section concerned.
(c) Recovery or improvement after removal of the posited cause (a difficult criterion to meet, but to be considered if the circumstances are relevant).
(d) No other obvious cause.

A list of the items concerned (other than those in Section 21 itself) is provided for ease of reference, as follows:

13.034	Dissociative
13.036	Anxiety
13.037	Obsessional
13.038	Depressive
13.043	Manic
20.061	Perceptual
20.062-064	Hallucinatory
20.065,066	First rank
20.067	Delusional
20.069	Catatonic

21.125 Identify organic cause for Section 21 symptoms

21.126 Interference of activities due to Section 21 symptoms

OPTIONAL CHECKLIST

21.127- 21.134 Mild cognitive disorder

The main symptoms of this disorder are stated as follows:

(a) Subjective forgetfulness for recent events (**21.127**) including ratings like those of (1) in **21.030 - 21.032**, but which cannot be attributed to inattention, worry, etc.;
(b) Poor concentration on tasks such as reading, writing or repetitive domestic or work tasks (**21.128**) indicated by ratings of (1) or (2) in **7.002**;
(c) Subjective difficulty in attempting new learning (**21.129**);
(d) a, b, and c were present for at least 2 weeks;
(e) There was evidence of infection or physical disorder either cerebral or systematic, concurrent with the symptoms or closely preceding or following them (**21.133**).
(f) Difficulty in thinking - problem-solving or abstraction (**21.130**).
(g) Language difficulties (**21.131**).
(h) Neuropsychological test decline.

22 Motor and behavioral items

GENERAL POINTS ABOUT SECTION 22

Ratings can be made of behavioral abnormalities observed during the interview or recorded from other sources during the previous month.

EXAMINATION FOR MOVEMENT DISORDERS

This examination is suitable for screening purposes only. It covers both psychiatric and neurological disorders and supplements the disorders of movement and speech (Sections 22 and 24) rated on the basis of the whole clinical examination. Finer detail will be provided in an associated instrument being prepared by WHO. Some of the following items, such as the first, can be taken at other points in the interview. Side effects of medication can be rated on the AIMS scale (NIMH, 1974) and the TAKE scale (Wojcik et al, 1980).

OBSERVE FACE, HEAD, NECK, TRUNK AND LIMBS DURING THE FOLLOWING EXERCISES FOR ABNORMALITIES OF POSTURE AND MOVEMENT

OFFER TO SHAKE HANDS

If an unusual reaction, consider: negativism, ambitendence, forced grasping, autistic spectrum.

FLEX AND EXTEND ELBOWS GENTLY

If unusual tone, consider: flexibilitas, spasticity, freezing.

ASK RESPONDENT TO STAND STILL

Consider akathisia.

ASK R TO EXTEND ARMS IN FRONT OF BODY, PALMS DOWN

Consider tremor, choreic movement, athetosis, posture, axial hyperkinesis.

ASK R TO TOUCH EXAMINER'S FINGER AND THEN OWN NOSE

Arm should be completely extended, i.e. examiner should stand sufficiently far away. Consider intention tremor.

ASK R TO IMITATE FACIAL MOVEMENTS AND EXPRESSION

Examiner should smile, frown, wink, blow out both cheeks. Consider ability to imitate facial expressions and rapidity of change from one to another. Consider facial immobility.

ASK R TO OPEN MOUTH AND PROTRUDE TONGUE

Consider facial and oral movement. Drooling. State of teeth and dentures.

ASK R TO WALK ACROSS ROOM THEN RETURN

Consider gait.

RATINGS OF BEHAVIOR, SPEECH AND AFFECT

Most items in Sections 22-24 are rated on a simple 3-point scale (0-2). The basis for rating is severity and frequency during the past month. Information from records or an informant should be used as well as observation during the interview. Severe behavioral abnormalities may not be observed at examination because of the short time sample, but when they are present skilled direct observations are of great importance. The items listed are also worth rating because of their possible juxtaposition with other symptoms.

The scale is built round a 0-1-2 format, because it is not anticipated that a broader range would be appropriate in the usual circumstances of the interview. As is the case with Rating Scale II, a rating of (1) meets the criterion for an item being 'present' for the purposes of the classifying algorithms in the CATEGO5 computer programs.

Difficulty may arise if it is thought that the item is present but is due to a drug or physical cause. If the presence of the item is in doubt rate 8. If the examiner is absolutely certain that what is observed is only due to a physical factor and remits on its withdrawal rate 9 (not applicable) and consider the need for rating attribution of cause in Section 20. If it is clear that the item is present, but its cause is less certain, rate the item as present and rate possible attribution of cause in Section 20.

Many behavioral items are also included in Item Groups and can be rated in the Checklist.

Always consider **21.065 - 21.087**, which are also behavioral items, if there is any possibility of cognitive impairment.

RATING SCALE III

0 This is a positive rating of absence. It does not mean 'not known' or 'uncertain whether present or not'. It can only be used if sufficient information is available to establish its accuracy.

1 Unequivocally present during past month, moderate severity only. Use all information available.

2 Present in severe form during past month or at examination.

8 If, after an adequate examination, the interviewer is still not sure whether a symptom is present (rated 1-3) or absent (rated 0), the rating is (8). This is the only circumstance in which (8) is used. It should not be used to indicate a mild form of the symptom or to record the absence of information.

9 This rating is only used if the information needed to rate an item is incomplete in some respect, for example because of language or cognitive disorder, or lack of co-operation, or because the interviewer did not complete the examination. It is distinguished from (8) because the examination could not be (or was not) carried out adequately. If due to physical factor rate (9).

REDUCED MOTOR ACTIVITY

22.001 Slumped posture

Take age into account when assessing this sign.

22.002 Stillness

Sits or stands abnormally still. Very little movement unless asked to move.

22.003 - 22.004 Slowness and underactivity

The subject walks and moves abnormally slowly or takes a long time to initiate movement. The symptom has to be fairly marked, and unusual for the subject. Rate (1) if it is not present continuously but there are periods of normal activity or overactivity. Rate (2) if the subject is retarded and underactive continuously.

If the retardation or underactivity is thought to be due to medication, rate (9) and specify.

Do not include if retardation is due to organic causes, peripheral or central (e.g. Parkinsonism) - rate (9) and specify.

22.005 Stupor

Total or nearly total lack of spontaneous movement and marked decrease in reactivity to environment.

22.006 Slow speech

There are long pauses before the subject answers and each word follows very slowly after the one before. Often the subject stops answering altogether and has to be reminded before starting again. The interview may be impossible to complete because the subject is so slow and cannot be hurried. Rate such severe slowness, shown continuously, as (2); less marked degrees of the symptom are rated as (1).

Do not include drawling or slow articulation. Always give the subject the benefit of any doubt concerning education, fluency and ability to use language. If in any doubt, rate the symptom as absent.

Differentiate from restricted quantity of speech (item **24.016**), which need not be associated with slowness of movement.

22.007 Shuffling gait

Take age into account when assessing this sign.

22.008 Arms not swung

USE OF NON-VERBAL MEANS OF COMMUNICATION

22.09 Negative posture

Rate aversion, whether passive, e.g. eyes closed, hunched, head bowed, etc. rate (1), or active, e.g. head turned away, avoids eye contact, back turned rate (2).

22.010 Gesture

Little use of gesture to accompany speech or illustrate meaning rate (1), or virtually no use of gesture at all rate (2).

22.011 Facial expression

Little change in expression to accompany or illustrate meaning or feeling rate (1), or virtually expressionless face giving no clue to inner thoughts or feelings rate (2).

22.012 Expression in voice

Voice changes little in expression with change of topic (rate 1), or voice monotonous and expressionless throughout speech rate (2).

22.013 Eye-contact

Eye contact used unskillfully, e.g. stares, gives wrong cues, etc. rate (1), or makes almost no eye contact at all or only inappropriate rate (2).

INCREASED MOTOR ACTIVITY

22.014 Distractibility

The respondent's attention is taken up by trivial events occurring while the interview proceeds which usually would not be noticed, let alone interfere with the interview. The respondent is unable to sustain attention for a period required by the task at hand. The subject may remark on the pattern of the wallpaper instead of replying to a question, or break off to comment on the furniture or the sound of someone walking by. If this is occurring continuously, rate (2). If it occurs quite markedly but not continuously, rate (1). Write down an example.

22.015 Restlessness

Purposeless movements of extremities, limbs; fiddling, stretching, shifting, cannot sit still, standing up and sitting down again.

A mild degree of fidgeting is common and should not be included. Larger movements with a background of anxiety should be rated at item **22.017**.

22.016 Agitation

This symptom consists of excessive motor movement with a background of marked anxiety. R cannot sit in a chair or lie down but paces up and down or has to stand up from time to time and possibly break off the interview because of motor restlessness.

Agitation is a severe symptom even when rated (1). Distinguish, however, from gross excitement (item **22.018**) in which the subject runs rather than walks, and is much wilder and perhaps more hostile. Also distinguish from stereotypies (item **22.049**) in which the subject repeats certain stereotyped movements such as rocking, rubbing, grimacing, etc.

22.017 Overactivity and excitement

R is wildly excited, running about the room, jumping, flinging arms about, perhaps shouting or screaming. R may throw things, or be aggressive. Rate (1) if intermittent or one brief episode after which R calms down and interview can continue. Rate (2) if more than one episode or if more continuous and subject cannot be interviewed because of the symptom.

Distinguish from agitation (item **22.017**) in which the subject is anxious rather than angry and is not aggressive, destructive or wild.

22.018   Rapid alternation between stupor and excitement

22.019   Destruction and violence

Rate destructiveness (1); violent behavior to people (2).

POSSIBLE CATATONIC BEHAVIOR

22.021 - 22.030   Catatonic symptoms

Catatonic movements are nowadays very rare. Do not rate them as present unless there is little doubt about them. If there is suspicion of organic disease, rate (9) and specify.

22.020   Negativism

Negativism occurs when the subject consistently does the opposite of what is asked, e.g. asked to open the hand, it is closed tighter.

22.021   Ambitendence

Ambitendence is fluctuation between two alternatives. R is unable to complete an intended movement. For example, when trying to pass through a door, R advances, withdraws, advances again, etc. Or R begins to take the hand the examiner proffers, then withdraws, then makes to take it again, and so on.

22.022   Forced grasping

R takes the examiner's hand repeatedly, or is unable to let go again.

22.023   Echopraxia and echolalia

R appears to imitate movements made by others, or echoes others' speech. Distinguish from delayed echolalia (item **24.024**).

22.024   Flexibilitas cerea

Flexibilitas cerea is a condition in which the muscles of a limb become fairly rigid and the arm, if moved passively, moves without jerking. If an arm is raised into a certain position the patient will hold it for at least fifteen seconds.

22.025 Opposition

Movement in any direction is countered by equal resistance in the opposite direction.

22.026 Jerkiness

Lack of smoothness of voluntary movement.

22.027 Freezing

Includes 'freezing' in one posture during voluntary movement.

22.028 Automatic obedience

Excessive co-operation in passive movement. R can be pushed into uncomfortable postures by finger-tip pressure from the examiner.

22.029 Catatonia dominant

Catatonic symptoms dominate the clinical picture.

22.030 Date/s of PERIOD/S of catatonic symptoms

22.031 Interference due to catatonic symptoms

22.032 Organic cause of catatonic symptoms

A simple rating of whether an 'organic' cause is present, whether or not it can be specified in terms of an ICD-10 class, can be made at **22.033** and in Section 20 at item **20.069**.

22.033 Identify the organic cause of catatonic symptoms

A range of organic conditions (for example, cerebral tumors and encephalitis) can be associated with catatonic symptoms. The letter identifying the ICD-10 chapter, and up to three digits, should be entered at etiology option here at **22.034** or at items **20.077, 20.079** or **20.081**. A list of ICD-10 categories is provided in the Appendix.

The effects of psychoactive substances, should be rated in Sections 11 or 12.

Dementias and other cognitive disorders are rated in Section 21.

ODD BEHAVIOR OR APPEARANCE

22.034 Odd or inappropriate appearance

Odd clothes, ornaments etc. Would look odd to most people because of posture, gait etc.

22.035 Embarrassing behavior

The subject makes sexual suggestions or advances to the interviewer. Does not show social restraint; belches or passes flatus loudly or scratches genitals, either without shame or without apparent concern for the conventions. If R's behavior is characterized in this way continuously, rate (2). Otherwise rate (1).

Do not include unpolished manners due to lack of social education. Do not include irreverent behavior (item **22.038**) but the two symptoms can be present together.

22.036 Bizarre appearance and behavior

This symptom is only rated on the basis of oddities of appearance that are clearly related to R's psychotic condition. For example, secret documents or codes, clothes or ornaments with a special significance (one lady wore a specially constructed hat `to keep the rays off'). Rate (1) or (2) if the whole impression is grossly odd and would be remarked on by a fairly unsophisticated person.

Do not include a mild degree of eccentricity or even a major degree if it is clearly determined by membership of a social sub-group. The main criterion is whether the odd appearance is determined by the subject's psychotic symptoms.

Do not include mannerisms or posturing which are rated at items **22.047** and **22.048**.

22.037 Irreverent behavior

The respondent sings, makes facetious remarks or silly jokes, is unduly familiar with strangers, does not observe ordinary social conventions. This behavior should be marked and unmistakable, even for a rating of (1). If it is present continuously and affects all situations which arise during it, rate (2). Write down an example.

Distinguish from socially embarrassing behavior (item **22.036**).

22.038 Histrionic behavior

R's feelings are expressed in an exaggerated, dramatic, histrionic manner. Rate (1) or (2) according to intensity and frequency.

22.040 - 22.052 Behavior associated with mental impairment

These items allow ratings of aspects of behavior associated with an inability to understand and follow ordinary conventions of social behavior. Many different disorders may be associated, including mild mental retardation, dementia, schizophrenia and disorders in the autistic spectrum, but all have this common theme. Each item has its own significance and should be rated independently of the others.

Only severe behavior disturbance should be considered. Therefore rate on the basis of frequency during the month, using information from informants and case records, as well as direct observation. Rate (9) if the behavior is probably or definitely due to an identifiable physical disease. If this disease is not identified in earlier Sections, enter it at items **27.083 - 27.088**.

22.039 Self-neglect

Consider R's degree of cleanliness, state of hair, make-up and clothes, whether shaven or not, etc. Only rate self-neglect if there is marked lack of attention to at least one of these aspects of personal appearance.

Take into account what opportunity R has had to take care of appearance - do not rate self-neglect because dressed in pajamas and unshaven, if there has been no opportunity to look otherwise. Also check whether nursing staff have taken special care to prevent self-neglect from showing rate (9).

Do not include simple untidiness. Self-neglect must be marked for it to be rated even (1). Rate (2) if R is markedly neglectful most of the time, or needs constant supervision to prevent it.

22.040 Neglect of health care

Consider diet, shelter, clothes, compliance with treatment for physical illnesses, dental hygiene.

22.041 Personal hygiene and habits

Include only markedly abnormal behavior such as spitting (apart from socially sanctioned habits), smearing faeces, eating rubbish, etc.

22.042 Self injury

Include head banging, picking sores, biting self, etc. Exclude self-harm in context of depression.

22.043 Creates chaos

Picks up and moves or throws objects, apparently at random. Literally creates chaos in an orderly environment.

22.044 Neglect of common dangers

Does not understand common dangers. Needs supervision because of risk from gas taps, fires, busy roads, etc.

22.045 Hoarding objects

Accumulates large quantities of useless objects, such as old newspapers and junk. May carry large quantities of objects of a particular kind, e.g. wrappers from packets of sweets. Shows distress if parted from them.

22.046 Complex mannerisms

Mannerisms are odd, stylized movements, usually specific to R and sometimes apparently suggestive of special meaning or purpose. For example, R may salute three times before entering a room or get up and walk round a chair from time to time or make complex gestures with the hands. Any apparent meaning, if recognized by the examiner, should not be taken into account when rating this item.

If the interview or recent history indicates the frequent occurrence of mannerisms, rate (2). Otherwise rate (1).

Do not include simple stereotypies (item **22.049**) in which R repeats stereotyped movements such as rocking, nodding or grimacing, which do not seem to have special significance.

22.047 Posturing

R assumes and maintains uncomfortable postures for 10 minutes to several hours at a time. Include unusual configurations of the limbs, or hand and fingers ('Balinese dancer' postures), or other local parts of the body, which would be very difficult for most people to sustain for long periods.

22.048 Simple stereotypies

R performs certain repetitive movements such as rocking to and fro on a chair, rubbing the head round and round with one hand, audible grinding of the teeth, nodding the head or grimacing. Include tics. These movements do not appear to have any special significance. If they continue more or less continuously, rate (2), otherwise rate (1).

Akathisia is rated (9), depending on cause, if it takes the form of a simple stereotypy.

Distinguish from agitation (item **22.017**) in which R is anxious, fidgeting and restless and may pace up and down but does not perform repetitive movements.

22.049 Inappropriate laughter or giggling

Rate laughter in circumstances where there is no evident justification for amusement in the emotional or social context. The examiner's judgement should be based on empathy with the respondent's frame of mind. Such laughter can be described as 'empty', since there is apparently no subjective affect. Behavior of this kind is sometimes regarded (like 'talking to oneself') as evidence for private hallucinatory experiences. However, the rating should be based only on the behavior observed and not on hypotheses about possible causes.

22.050 Apparently hallucinating behavior

A presumption that R is auditorily hallucinated might be made from behavior such as that rated at item **22.051**. R's lips move soundlessly; R looks round as though voices might be calling; R says something unintelligible that might be an answer. These signs do not necessarily indicate hallucinations and should not be regarded, in themselves, as evidence. Distinguish also the champing movements of the mouth which are often present in people with brain damage and those who have been for a long time on phenothiazine medication.

If the behavior is continuous throughout the interview, rate (2), otherwise rate (1). If there is a known organic cause, rate (9), including side-effects of medication.

22.051 Behavior associated with a single interest

Behavior of this kind is usually obvious if a description (which R can often, but not always give) is available from an informant. R's sole interest may be in railway timetables, in the classification of a particular species of bird, or the day of the week on which dates of past or future events fall. This interest is based on rote learning. It is not scholarly, or part of an investigation with some wider purpose. It is stereotyped, rigid, and unmodifiable, and it excludes many activities necessary for everyday functioning. The people affected are usually severely disabled socially.

23 Affect

The affects rated in Section 23, if present, will have been displayed during the interview, or convincingly described by informants or in case records as present during the previous month. They are rated using Scale III.

23.001 Observed anxiety

R has a tense or worried look or posture; may look and sound fearful or apprehensive. There may be a tremor of voice or hands, tachycardia or other evidence of autonomic anxiety. If R definitely shows anxiety more or less continuously, rate (2), otherwise rate (1). Be critical about the threshold of rating. There has to be a fairly marked degree of anxiety present (taking into account that the examination itself may be somewhat anxiety provoking for some people) for the symptoms to be rated present at all.

23.002 Observed depression

Rate a sad, mournful look with tears in eyes and gloomy monotonous voice, as (1). If R's voice chokes on distressing topics, there are frequent deep sighs and tears, rate (2). Also include 'frozen misery', if examiner is sure that it is present, as (2).

23.003 Observed elation

R is moderately elated, unduly smiling and cheerful irrespective of context, but the good humor may readily turn to irritability. Rate this condition (1). If R becomes highly elated or exalted rate (2).

23.004 Hostile irritability

Rate (1) if R is uncooperative, irritable, prickly, discontented or antagonistic. Rate (2) if R is angry or overtly hostile or if the interview has to be discontinued because of irritability.

Exclude gross excitement (items **22.018, 22.020**) - in which R becomes wild and may actually attack people or destroy things. The two symptoms can, of course, be present together.

23.005 Perplexity

R looks puzzled and cannot provide any explanation for unusual experiences. These may be delusions of reference, perceptual changes, intruded thoughts, etc., or R may simply be disoriented. Rate (1) or (2) according to the severity and duration of the symptom also during the interview.

Perplexity may co-exist with suspiciousness (item **22.010**), particularly when R is not clear about the reasons for suspicion, only that there is something to be suspicious about. The two symptoms are quite separate, however, and should be rated independently. Consciousness is clear.

23.006 Lability of mood

R's mood is changeable, at one moment frightened, at another confident. Euphoria may alternate with depression or hostility with friendliness. Include different degrees of manifestation of one mood, e.g. fluctuations between normal cheerfulness and elation. All these variants are included, i.e. consider only the changeability of the mood, not what type of mood is present. Rate (1) or (2) according to the frequency of change and briefness of stable moods.

23.007 Emotional outbursts

Rate the uncontrolled manifestation of moods of any kind. The most usual is anger, but fear or excitement are also common. The rating is based on the frequency and intensity of the outbursts.

23.008 Blunted affect

This term includes flatness of affect, emotional indifference and apathy. Essentially, the symptom involves a global diminution of emotional response. R's face and voice are expressionless, there is no involvement with the interview or emotional response to changing topics of conversation. Apparently distressing matters are met with apparent indifference when discussed (whether or not delusional). There is a very limited range of emotional expression. If severe and fairly uniform continuously, very little rapport, and almost no emotional response, with expressionless face and monotonous voice - rate (2). If severe but less uniform continuously, or less marked though uniform, rate (1).

Differentiate from incongruity of affect (item **23.009**), in which affect is expressed but is not in keeping with the affect which would ordinarily be expected to accompany the concurrent thought process.

Make this rating independently of any diagnostic formulation (this is true of all ratings in the PSE but particularly of this one). A depressed person may have a limited range of emotional expression while someone with schizophrenia has a normal range, as well as vice versa.

23.009 Incongruity of affect

The range of emotional expression is not necessarily diminished (it may even be increased) but the emotion experienced(and often expressed) is not in keeping with that expected to accompany the concurrent thought process. For example, R may laugh when discussing a sad event. If this sort of incongruity occurs only a few times, rate (1). If it occurs more frequently, rate (2).Differentiate from mere inappropriate affect.

Do not rate a simple failure to show emotion when expected as incongruity but as blunting (item **23.008**).

23.010 Suspiciousness

R expresses the feeling that everything is not as it should be - this is clear from what is said about relations with other people and with the environment during the past month. Usually R thinks that there may be a deliberate attempt to harm or annoy, beyond what the circumstances would warrant (clearly some people might be suspicious with justification - only pathological suspicion should be rated). If R does show suspicion in this sense but is not openly suspicious of the interview procedure, rate (1). If R also seems to think that the interviewer, or some part of the interview procedure, is itself part of the process, rate (2).

Distinguish from puzzlement, in which the respondent does not apparently suspect a particular kind of cause (e.g. a plot or attempt to annoy) but simply does not know how to explain what is going on (item **23.005**). Remember, however, that some people may attempt to conceal the reason for their suspicions.

24 Speech abnormalities

GENERAL POINTS ON SECTION 24 ITEMS

Three types of disordered **content of speech** are specified: incoherence (item **24.012**), flight of ideas (item **24.005**) and poverty of content (**24.015**). These are overlapping concepts and, in each case, the effect is to make it difficult to grasp what the subject means. However, the symptoms are defined in terms of specific components so that it should, in most cases, be possible to say whether one, two or all three symptoms are present. If in doubt, rate hierarchically, i.e. rate incoherence in preference to flight of ideas and flight of ideas in preference to poverty of speech.

If the patient does not talk enough to give a rateable sample of speech, rate all three symptoms (9).

Always give the respondent the benefit of any doubt concerning education, fluency and ability to use language.

24.001 Abnormal loudness of voice

24.002 Abnormal quietness of voice

These two symptoms should be rated on the extent to which they are markedly and often embarrassingly inappropriate to the social context. Loudness is likely to be more noticeable than quietness. If an abnormally quiet voice is due to physical impairments, such as Parkinson's syndrome, rate (9).

24.003 Mumbling 'to self'

Include whispering, muttering and mumbling 'to self', without audible words, and soundless lip movements, that occur independently of the social context. The attribution 'to self' is misleading, since it implies that R is holding a normal two-way conversation 'with self'. The essence of the behavior to be rated is non-social verbigeration, carried on without regard for the social context, so that it appears markedly odd.

If words can be made out, rate also at item **24.022**.

24.004 Pressure of speech

R talks too much, there seems to be undue pressure to get the words out, he speaks too fast, the voice is too loud and unnecessary words are added. Speech is spontaneous and there is a difficulty in interrupting the respondent. If this is continuous, rate (2). If only some periods of speech are characterized in this way, or if only some of the elements are evident but not others (though the whole impression is definitely abnormal), rate (1).

24.005 Flight of ideas

Words are associated together inappropriately because of their meaning or rhyme (white-black-coffin, splash-hash-fascist, ring-wrong). R is easily distracted, so that speech loses its aim and wanders far from the original theme. One respondent, seeing another patient walking past the window said, '*She is going for ECT. Etcetera treatment or teddy-bear's picnic, I call it*'. There is frequent punning.

If the whole conversation is of this kind, so that it is difficult to conduct a useful conversation all, rate (2). If flight of ideas is marked but it is still possible to grasp some of R's meaning, rate (1). Always write down a sample of the speech.

Differentiate from `knight's move' in which it is very difficult to see how the change in topic comes about (item **24.012**).

24.006 Circumstantiality

Gets lost in insignificant detail. Cannot differentiate what is essential and therefore loses the thread of the answer. Gives far more detail about some particular topic (or fragment of a topic) than is necessary.

24.007 Rambling speech

'Drivelling' or rambling in a vague, muddled way, beginning more or less on the point but gradually wandering far from it. The overall effect, after some time, is one of incoherence but short sections of speech may appear within normal limits. Distinguish from **24.006** (because R wanders from subject); **24.011** (see definition) and **24.014** (because some information may be given).

24.008 Perseveration

Words or phrases repeated so as to be meaningless. Extreme form is verbigeration, rated (2). Distinguish from item **21.080**, which occurs in a context of cognitive impairment.

24.009 Rumination

Endless preoccupation with one theme. Mulling over a topic to no purpose. This is the representation in speech of item **5.006**.

24.010 Approximate answers

R understands the point of the question and answers in a related but incorrect way, e.g. gives a completely wrong date or place: '*What's your address?*'. '*It's supposed to be Salisbury near Birmingham.*'

24.011 Neologisms and idiosyncratic use of words or phrases

R uses words that are made up and have no generally accepted meaning, as in the following example:

'One is called Per-God and the other is called Per-the-Devil ... miracle-willed through God's Tarn-harn. Well, there is a frequenting of clairvoyance ...'

`Per-God`, `Per-the-Devil`, and `Tarn-harn` are neologisms.

Only gross and bizarre use of words or phrases, equivalent in effect to neologisms, should be rated, e.g. `miracle-willed`, `frequenting of clairvoyance`. Ordinary idiosyncrasies should not be included. Make due allowance for lack of education or intelligence.

Rate (1) if only a few examples. Rate (2) if whole conversation is interlarded with examples.

Always write down the evidence for the rating.

24.012 Incoherence of speech

R's grammar is distorted (e.g. `They've all been going he she first wife'),  or grossly pedantic phrases obscure the meaning, or there are unexplained shifts from topic to topic (`knight's move'), or there is a lack of logical connection between one part of a sentence and another or between one sentence and the next. This is also referred to as formal thought disorder. For example:

'We've seen the downfall of the radium crown by the Roman Catholics, whereas when you come to see the drinking side of the business, God saw that Noah, if he lost his reason, he got nobody there to look after them.'

'I did suggest to you, that intrinsic or congenital sentiment or refinement of disposition would be so miracle-willed through God's `tarn-harn' as to assume quite the opposite.'

'I believe we live in a world, in an age, where the elements are a force that elders of professionalism hope, not to conquer, but to control.'

If R's speech is completely incoherent, as in these three examples, rate (2). A lesser degree of incoherence, so that some of R's meaning does get through, is rated (1).

Note that a free flow of speech interlarded with bizarre delusions is not necessarily incoherent. R may talk about delusions with great precision and coherence.

Always make due allowance for poor education, poor intelligence or poor grasp of the language. Always write down an example.

Differentiate from item **24.005**, flight of ideas, where a movement from one theme to another is fairly easy to follow because of clang associations or associations of the white-black-coffin variety. `Knight's move' is a totally unexpected switch of topic, with no link apparent (or only a sophisticated interpretation can make sense of it). The two symptoms can be present together but are very difficult to isolate from each other. If so, rate the identifiable component as present and rate the other (8).

24.013 Magical or markedly illogical thinking

24.014 Blocking

Blocking is sudden interruption in a line of speech without recognizable reason, so that R stops in the middle of a sentence and cannot recapture the theme. It is not distraction, lapse of attention, or lack of understanding. R stops talking and then begins again on same or different topic.

24.015 Poverty of content of speech

R talks fairly freely but so vaguely that no information is given, in spite of the number of words used. This symptom may appear to be readily recognizable in some of one's colleagues, therefore only rate it when it is really pathological. The following example would be rated (2).

Q. `*How do you like it in hospital?*'

A. `*Well, er ... not quite the same as, er...don't know quite how to say it. It isn't the same, being in hospital as, er...working, er...the job isn't quite the same, er ... very much the same but, of course, it isn't exactly the same.*'

Include also examples of frequent repetitiveness or perseveration. These would usually be rated as (1).

Always make due allowance for poor education or intelligence or use of language. Always write down a sample of speech by way of example.

24.016 Restricted quantity of speech

R repeatedly fails to answer, questions have to be repeated, answers are restricted to the minimum (often one word, or telegrammatic style). Rate this condition (2). If R answers readily enough but only with the minimum necessary number of words, and does not use extra sentences or unprompted additional comments, so that it is extremely difficult to keep a conversation going, rate (1).

For example:

Q. `What work do you do?'
A. `I'm a machinist. I work at Simpson's.' Pause, then without prompting: `It's a decent sort of job really.'

`I work at Simpson's' is an extra sentence. `It's a decent sort of job really' is an unprompted additional comment.

Differentiate from slowness of speech (item **22.007**) which is usually normal speech slowed down so that the examiner samples rather few words. Restricted quantity does not necessarily imply slowness. The two symptoms can, however, appear together.

Always write down an example.

24.017 Muteness

Rate (1) if R is almost mute, and says no more than twenty words in answer to questions, including introductory section. (Do not include non-social speech when making a rough assessment of number of words used. A `mute' respondent may talk a lot outside the context of the interview).

Rate (2) if R utters no more than half a dozen recognizable words in answer to questions throughout the interview.

24.018 Nonverbal communication during speech

Lack or under-use of normal non-verbal gestures, facial expressions, changes of tone and pitch and loudness, eye-contact etc., during conversation.

24.019 Ability to keep conversation going

No small talk. Does not initiate or keep a conversation going.

24.020 Rewards in conversation

R does not reward the other person for speaking by non-verbal acknowledgements, nodding, smiling, 'I see', etc. For example, R may conduct a monologue, with no understanding of taking turn' in conversation. Items **22.010 - 22.014, 24.019** and **24.024** may co-exist but are rated independently.

24.021 Misleading answers

R answers at random, or answers `Yes' to all questions, or frequently contradicts himself, or appears to be deliberately misleading. If marked, so that it is difficult to trust any of the ratings made, rate (2). If only some of the replies seem to be misleading, rate (1).

24.022 Non-social speech

Non-social speech, some words of which are clearly audible, but which quite clearly does not fit within the social context of the interview, i.e. is not addressed to the examiner in answer to questions or as part of the conversation. Irrelevant or incoherent replies to or comments on the examiner's questions are counted as social, not non-social, speech. Include talking to self' spontaneously or trailing on after a question has been answered, and shouting `to voices', so long as the words can be heard. Rate mumbling or muttering or soundless lip movements at item **24.003**.

Rate (1) if definitely present but not a marked feature. Rate (2) if a marked feature (in which case the interview is likely to be incomplete).

Do not rate non-social speech as present unless it clearly fits the definition. If in doubt, exclude it. Always give the respondent the benefit of any doubt concerning education, fluency and ability to use language.

24.023 Grossly pedantic speech

Over-formal, over-technical terms or phrases that sound odd in ordinary conversation and are used without understanding that they are inappropriate. For example, a hole in a sock was referred to as '*a temporary absence of knitting*'. A man said to his mother, '*and how is the foetus today?*' Asked what he would like for tea, he said, '*I elect to extract a biscuit from the tin.*' These were not attempts to be facetious but incorrect imitations of normal speech.

Include only examples of speech with this degree of abnormality. Exclude ordinary pomposity of phrasing.

24.024 Repetitive speech and delayed echolalia

R talks on one theme regardless of attempts to widen the scope of the conversation. This may take the form of repetitive questioning of the interviewer, which continues whatever answers are given, or it may center on R's circumscribed interests (item **22.049**). Delayed echolalia is the frequent stereotyped repetition of one or more phrases, often copied directly from other people, using the same words, with the same intonation, each time. The phrases, when copied, may include reversal of pronouns, for example; '*Do you want a cup of tea?*' is echoed exactly, but means '*I want a cup of tea*'.

24.025 Ungrammatical speech in real attempt to communicate

24.026 Made-up words in real attempt to communicate

These abnormalities result when adult respondents with impairments such as those evident in delayed echolalia attempt to use speech to communicate. For example, *'I did went on bus'*. Made-up words are similar in origin. For example, *'tram-bus'* for trolley-bus, *'earring plugs'* for headphones, *'gas-lectric dishpyer'* for dishwasher. These examples are unlikely to be mistaken, in adults, for lack of education.

24.027 No 'theory of mind'

R's behavior and speech indicate an impairment of the ability to see through other people's eyes; to put oneself into their position and experience in imagination their outlook and emotions. The problem is not deliberate selfishness but a lack of awareness that other people have thoughts, ideas and feelings with a resulting innocent egocentricity. For example, a young man expected to receive birthday presents from others but was completely unable to understand that he should spend some of his money on presents for others.

24.028 Evasiveness

R avoids answering direct questions about symptoms, particularly those with an embarrassing connotation. Use Scale III. Do not rate misleading answers here but at item **24.021**.

24.029 - 24.031 Note the rating scales

These four items have rating scales with a range from 0-3. Do not use Scale III.

24.029 Lack of direction or purpose

Rate this item on the whole interview and other information available. Consider evidence of motivation and initiative, active interests, plans for the future.

24.030 Insight into positive Part Two symptoms

Take into account the explanations given by R for symptoms rated present in Part Two of PSE10, and the behavior associated with subjective symptoms.

24.031 Adequacy of ratings in Sections 22-24

This item should be carefully rated, taking into account two kinds of problem listed below. (These apply also to items **13.129, 20.092, 27.059**). The effect of such problems can be to limit the examiner's ability to explore the phenomena appropriately through the process of clinical cross-examination and thus limit the accuracy of the ratings made.

The number of items rated (8) is provided as a separate score for each Item Group in the output from SCAN. This overall adequacy rating will also be an important factor in assessing the value of the output.

Sources of information

- Language problems rated in Section 15.
- Abnormalities of speech rated in Section 24.
- Poor cooperation during the interview.
- Evasiveness, rated at **24.028**.
- Poor quality of information from case records or informants.

Rater's own problems

- Inadequate knowledge of language or dialect (R's and that of records and informants).
- Lack of familiarity with R's culture, social class, etc.
- Lack of clinical experience.
- Lack of training in SCAN techniques.

25   Social impairment

GENERAL POINTS ABOUT SECTION 25

This Section should be used if the interview as a whole, and items **24.023 - 24.027** in particular, suggest the presence of social impairment. See also items **27.029 - 27.033**. Use information gathered at interview, from informants, or from records. The period covered is the past month. Leave blank if not completed.

The term 'social impairment', as used in the present context, refers to a disorder of the understanding and use of the subtle rules of social interaction and social empathy. It is manifested in behavior that is odd, unusual and abnormal in any social context and for any chronological age or level of intellectual ability. For example, the behavior is markedly outside the limits of normal variation in styles of dress and behavior with age, occupation and culture. It would be seen as odd in any culture.

Someone with this kind of impairment does not choose to be different or to challenge social conventions. The problem is a lack of intuitive understanding of how to fit into the social conventions of one's particular culture. Thus social impairment must be distinguished from anti-social behavior, which is observed in someone who does have understanding of social rules and of the consequences of breaking them.

The items in Section 25 are adapted from the Asperger Screening Questionnaire of Ehlers, Gillberg and Wing (1989). Examples from actual case histories have been added in order to emphasize the extreme nature of the behaviors that are to be rated in the Section.

25.001   Markedly stiff, over-formal, stilted manner

Manner is inappropriate to the social situation. For example, R stands upright, as if 'to attention', even in an informal group, or may offer to shake hands with an acquaintance on each occasion of frequent meetings during the same day.

25.002   Regarded as very eccentric by peers

The odd social manner, peculiarities of dress, behavior, interests, life style, or content or style of speaking, lead peers to regard R as very eccentric. For example, one young man wore bicycle clips on his trousers at all times of the day, not only when cycling. He became angry and abusive if the morning weather forecast did not exactly predict the weather during the day. His ambition was to live in a country where it was always snowing or always sunny. (He did not mind which).

25.003   Odd attachment to one or a few particular objects

The objects may be carried round with R even when inappropriate. For example, R insists on carrying a very large, battered suitcase everywhere, containing a collection of out-of-date railway timetables, although it can no longer be fastened and has to be held with both hands to prevent it falling open.

25.004 Wishes to be sociable but fails

R is unable to make relationships with peers; always on the edge of his or her social group, watching the interaction but unable to join in. R makes inappropriate approaches, for example asking embarrassing personal questions of strangers. Peers find R's social manner too naive and immature to be acceptable, although they feel sorry for him or her.

25.005 Can only cope with company on his/her own terms

For example, R is distressed if he stays in a social group of more than three people and has to go away to be alone every few minutes. Another R can only tolerate being with another person if he can talk on his favorite topic - the makes of aircraft that fly over his house and the statistics showing the differential likelihood of their crashing.

25.006 Has no real friend

Rate only if the problem arises from R's inability to understand the concept of friendship and the reciprocal sharing of ideas and feelings that this involves. It may be manifested in a complete lack of interest in others and a solitary lifestyle. Another respondent may want friends and ask for a set of rules to follow, but then follows them by rote, without understanding the consequent lack of success.

25.007 Lacks empathy

R fails to show sympathetic understanding when others are in pain and does not share their moments of pleasure or happiness. R does not seek comfort when in distress, or use physical gestures of empathy, such as shuddering with horror, smiling or grimacing appropriately during conversation.

25.008 Has little or no idea of how to work in a team

R may score 'own goals' due to lack of understanding of the conventional nature of the rules of a game, or of how to cooperate and interact with other people to achieve a target.

25.009 Conspicuously lacks common sense

R read in a newspaper that exercise increases physical fitness. He at once stripped to his underwear and ran several miles in the snow until he collapsed and was brought home by the police.

25.010 Clumsy, poorly coordinated, odd, ungainly movements

One respondent stands with head bowed, elbows flexed and hands drooping at the wrists. He walks without swinging his arms or with one swinging and the other held stiff. Another walks bent forward almost at a right angle, or lifting the feet very high at each step. There are no set patterns.

25.011 Tends to be exploited or bullied

R tends to be bullied at school because other children recognize his oddness. His naivety and vulnerability can be exploited. One respondent in search of friends became attached to a delinquent gang and was the only one to be caught because he did not understand the signal to run away.

25.012 Lives in a world of his/her own

Intensely preoccupied with a few idiosyncratic interests and cannot cope with everyday matters. One respondent lived in a house on his own and collected glass jars from dustbins. He had no other interest, did no housework; everything in the house was filthy except for hundreds of clean and shining jars. Another respondent spent all her time listening to records of classical music. Her mother had to ensure that she washed, dressed and ate, and that she attended to the other essentials of life.

25.013 Surprisingly good at a few isolated subjects

One respondent was poor at school work but an excellent chess player. Another was able to play exactly, by ear, any music after one hearing, with full harmony and variations. Another, whose daily life had to be organized for her in detail by her family, was a good computer programmer.

25.014 Accumulates facts without understanding them

Has a good rote memory but does not understand the meaning or make use of the knowledge. For example, one respondent knows, by rote from books, the names and nesting habits of all European birds but takes no interest whatever in birds that she sees around her. Another knows the day of the week on which any date in the past century falls. He asks everyone he meets the date of their marriage (even if they are single, and even if he has asked them many times before) in order to exercise his skill. Another knows the flight numbers and times of all planes and all airlines. He buys timetables and keeps up to date but makes no use of the information.

25.015 Odd style of communication, 'robotic', pedantic

R has a formal, fussy, pedantic or robot like language. He and his family have a marked local accent, but most of his speech is in the style of a formal radio announcer, using phrases copied from the weather forecast such as, '*A depression centered on the Northeast will bring cloud and a little light rain*'.

25.016 Fails to adjust speech to fit social context

R does not take account of the interests of different listeners, but takes every opportunity, however inappropriate, to give a list of all the records she owns. Another respondent will talk only about the history of the British police force, as obtained from one particular book. Whatever the audience, nothing will divert his monologue.

25.017 Makes naive and embarrassing remarks

One respondent comments loudly on the appearance of any passer-by who has a physical peculiarity. Another, regardless of the company and topic of conversation, insists on airing her decidedly eccentric views about artificial insemination.

25.018 Marked impairment of non-verbal means of expression

For example, R does not make eye contact during conversation, shows no facial expression, uses no gestures, does not nod or shake head in agreement or disagreement, and has a monotonous voice. Another respondent makes use of large, flailing gestures with no correspondence to what she is saying. Another has a vocal intonation that changes markedly from high to low.

26 Item group checklist

GENERAL POINTS ABOUT THE IGC

The Item Group Checklist (IGC) provides a simple means of rating information obtained only from case-records and/or informants other than the respondent. The IGs are not diagnostic syndromes; they cannot be translated directly into ICD-10 disorders but must be processed by a version of the CATEGO5 program adapted from the one that is applied to data from PSE10. The resulting classification is approximate compared with that from the PSE but it is a useful supplement to PSE information, and can substitute in situations where the PSE cannot be fully completed.

The 40 Item Groups included in the Checklist cover disorders in sub-chapters F2 (psychotic disorders), F3 (affective disorders) and F40-42 (neurotic disorders) of ICD-10. Disorders in sub-chapters F0 (cognitive impairment), F1 (substance use disorders), F43-45 (stress, dissociative and somatoform disorders) and F5 (appetite and sleep disorders and sexual dysfunctions), which are difficult to rate without interviewing or examining the respondent, are not included. It may occasionally be appropriate (particularly for the eating and substance use disorders) to rate the PSE itself from case-records or an informant.

Users of the IGC must have been trained in the use of the PSE and its Glossary, and be completely familiar with the structure of SCAN. This provides a substantial degree of operationalization for rating IGs, each of which is composed of designated PSE10 items.

INDICATIONS FOR USE

There are three main indications for using the IGC:

1   When the Respondent can provide information about present state but is unable or unwilling to remember or describe accurately the events or symptoms of a previous episode. In such a case, the previous period (RE or LB) is chosen and dated in the same way as for the PSE. However, it is not necessary, for most purposes, to use IGC to rate a past episode if the symptoms then were very similar to those in the present state.

2   When an interview with the respondent is impossible. In this case, the examiner chooses and dates PS, or PS + RE or PS + LB. The period/s chosen will depend on a clinical judgement as to which will most adequately cover the history. Both periods can be rated with IGC if no other method is possible. Often there will be an opportunity to observe behavior, speech and affect on examination, even when an interview is impossible. These observations can be used, with other information, to rate **26.048 [IG 31] - 26.057 [IG 40]**.

3   For use in research projects that require the maximum use of information in case records. Even when two PSEs have been completed, extra IGCs can be processed separately as a supplement to the routine package. Also, up to 6 episodes can be rated using PSEs, IGCs, or a mixture of the two.

THE STRUCTURE OF IGs AND RATING SCALE IV

Ratings of Item Groups should be entered in fixed format on the coding sheets, in the Record Book, or directly into the boxes provided in the SCAN schedule (including the laptop version).

The items themselves are not rated. They are listed in the IGC with their numbers and names in order to provide a general guide to the IG content. They are identical with items in the PSE10 text and the Glossary definitions are the same. The PSE10 criteria for presence and severity should be used as models when considering how to rate each IG. The threshold for rating a symptom present should be at least as high as that set in the PSE for the relevant item. If the quality of information is low, the threshold should be set even higher. These levels are specified against each item and raters are expected to be familiar with their clinical meaning as defined in PSE10. If in doubt, rate (8).

The guide to rating points in Scale IV provided on the next page should be interpreted in the light of the information available. Having considered the items making up each IG, make a global judgement as to how to rate the IG overall.

Each Item Group is given an overall rating based on the number of constituent symptoms present during the period and the severity of the distress or disablement that accompanies them. Clinical judgement is required in all cases, because the information will often be scanty. In addition, the criteria for rating must sometimes be relaxed on clinical grounds. For example, IG7 (**26.024**) is composed of five types of obsessional symptoms, but any one of them can be totally disabling (therefore rate 2). And if one type is present, and associated with only moderate disablement, it is still proper to give a rating of (1). The instructions for rating must be interpreted with clinical common sense.

A count of the number of IGs rated (8) (unsure whether present or absent) forms part of the output. Free use should be made of this rating, for example if the presence of psychotic or 'physical' symptoms make the rating of non-psychotic IGs difficult.

Since the information will sometimes be scanty, it is important to follow the general SCAN rule: 'When in doubt, choose the less definite or less severe rating'; (0) rather than (8), (8) rather than (1), (1) rather than (2).

It would occasionally be possible, if informants or case records were able to provide sufficient information, to score the IGs by rating each constituent symptom. This practice is not recommended, since in such a case the ratings would more easily be entered using the PSE.

RATING SCALE IV

0   This is a positive rating of absence. It does not mean 'not known' or 'uncertain whether present or not'. It can only be used if sufficient information is available to establish its accuracy.

1   Subject to clinical discretion, at least two items should definitely pass PSE threshold level, PLUS at least moderate disability (interference with everyday activities) and/or moderate or severe distress resulting from the symptoms.

2   As (1), but with severe degree of distress and/or disability. Usually at least three items pass PSE threshold but this is at the interviewer's clinical discretion.

8   If, after considering reasonably complete information, the interviewer is still not sure whether a symptom is present (rated 1 or 2) or absent (rated 0), the rating entered should be (8). This is the only circumstance in which (8) is used. It should not be used to indicate a mild form of the symptom or to record the absence of information.

9   This rating is only used if the information needed to rate an item is incomplete in some respect, for example because of gaps in the respondent's or an informant's account of the history, or the absence of case records. It is distinguished from (8) because the IGC could not be rated adequately.

26.059 Adequacy of ratings in IGC

This item should be carefully rated, taking into account two kinds of problem listed below. (These apply also to items **13.129, 20.092, 24.031**). The effect of such problems can be to limit the examiner's ability to explore the phenomena appropriately through the process of clinical cross-examination and thus limit the accuracy of the ratings made.

The number of items rated (8) is provided as a separate score for each Item Group in the output from SCAN. This overall adequacy rating will also be an important factor in assessing the value of the output.

Sources of information

- Language problems rated in Section 15.
- Abnormalities of speech rated in Section 23.
- Poor co-operation during the interview.
- Evasiveness, rated at **24.028**.
- Poor quality of information from case records or informants.

Rater's own problems

- Inadequate knowledge of language or dialect (R's and that of records and informants).
- Lack of familiarity with R's culture, social class, etc.
- Lack of clinical experience.
- Lack of training in SCAN techniques.

27 Clinical history schedule

The items in the CHS are mostly self-explanatory. They are completed from information from informants, records and the respondent. A detailed introduction to the CHS is provided in the SCAN text. This Section should not be overlooked in cases where a diagnosis of schizophrenia is considered a possibility as a number of ratings of social and occupational deficit are required for certain classification systems.

Several of the items involve a rating of 'average' performance (rating of 2). This is defined by local expectation, with which the rater must be familiar in order to make a judgement. The rating depends on an approximate comparison, in the first place, with people thought to be talented or competent beyond what is usual locally (rating of 1), or whether the respondent performs at a lower than average level. If the latter, a further decision is made as to whether performance is low but still within the range of ordinary expectations (rating of 3), or markedly lower than this (rating of 4).

These principles apply to items **27.002** and **27.025 - 27.039**.

The rest of the items in the CHS require clinical decisions. It is not expected that these can be more than approximate unless based on more detailed instruments, but the information should nevertheless be of value, both for research purposes (for example in the study of co-morbidity within cultures) and to develop hypotheses concerning cultural differences.

27.070 Quality of SCAN data

This item should be carefully rated, taking into account two kinds of problem listed below. (These apply also to items **13.129, 20.092, 24.031, 26.059**). The effect of such problems can be to limit the examiner's ability to explore the phenomena appropriately through the process of clinical cross-examination and thus limit the accuracy of the ratings made.

The number of items rated (8) is provided as a separate score for each Item Group in the output from SCAN. This overall adequacy rating will also be an important factor in assessing the value of the output.

Sources of information

- Language problems rated in Section 15.
- Abnormalities of speech rated in Section 24.
- Poor co-operation during the interview.
- Evasiveness, rated at **24.028.**
- Poor quality of information from case records or informants.

Rater's own problems

- Inadequate knowledge of language or dialect (R's and that of records and informants).
- Lack of familiarity with R's culture, social class, etc.
- Lack of clinical experience.
- Lack of training in SCAN techniques.

References:

American Psychiatric Association (1987) Diagnostic and statistical manual of mental disorders. Third edition-revised. Washington, DC: APA.

Bebbington P (1990) Continuity of development: PSE9 and PSE10. In: Stefanis CN (Ed.) Psychiatry. A World perspective. pp 93-99. Amsterdam: Elsevier.

Bebbington PE, Hurry J, Tennant C, Sturt E and Wing JK (1981) Epidemiology of mental disorders in Camberwell. Psychological Medicine 11: 561-580.

Brugha TS, Wing JK, Brewin CR, MacCarthy B, Mangen S, Lesage A and Mumford J (1988) The problems of people in long-term psychiatric day-care. An introduction to the Camberwell High Contact Survey. Psychological Medicine 18: 443-456.

Carpenter WT, Heinrichs DW, and Wagman AMI (1988). Deficit and non-deficit forms of schizophrenia: The concept. American Journal of Psychiatry 145:578-583

Cooper JE, Kendell RE, Gurland BJ, Sharpe L, Copeland JRM and Simon R (1972) Psychiatric diagnosis in New York and London. London: Oxford University Press.

Ehlers S, Gillberg C and Wing LG (1989) Social, communication and behavioral impairments and restrictive interests. Asperger syndrome. University of Gothenberg, Child Neuropsychiatry Center. Unpublished.

Isaac M (1990) SCAN in the Third World. In: Stefanis CN (ed) Psychiatry. A world perspective. pp 118-120. Amsterdam: Elsevier.

Holmes N, Shah A and Wing L (1982) The Disability Assessment Schedule. A brief screening device for use with the mentally retarded. Psychological Medicine 12: 897-890.

Jablensky A, Sartorius N, Hirschfeld R and Pardes H (1983) Diagnosis and classification of mental disorders and alcohol- and drug-related problems. A research agenda for the 1980s. Psychological Medicine 13:907-921.

Mavreas V (1990) Diagnosing dementias with the SCAN. In: Stefanis CN (ed) Psychiatry. A world perspective. pp 113-117. Amsterdam: Elsevier.

NIMH (1974) Abnormal Involuntary Movements Scale. Public Health Service: Bethesda, Maryland.

Robins LN, Wing JK, Wittchen H-U, Helzer J, Babor TF, Burke J, Farmer A, Jablensky A, Pickens R, Regier DA, Sartorius N and Towle LH (1988) The Composite International Diagnostic Interview. Archives of General Psychiatry 45:1069-1077.

Tomov T and Nikolov V (1990) Reliability of SCAN categories and scores. Results of the field trials. In: Stefanis CN (ed) Psychiatry. A world perspective. pp 107-112. Amsterdam: Elsevier.

Üstün TB (1990) SCAN: ICD-10 and DSM-III-R diagnoses. In: Stefanis CN (ed) Psychiatry. A world perspective. pp 100-106. Amsterdam: Elsevier.

Wing JK (1976) A technique for studying psychiatric morbidity in in-patient and out-patient series and in general population samples. Psychological Medicine 6, 665-671.

Wing JK (1983) Use and misuse of the PSE. British Journal of Psychiatry 143: 111-117.

Wing JK (1985) Methods of validation of psychiatric diagnosis and classification. In: Mental disorders, alcohol- and drug-related problems. Amsterdam: Exerpta Medica/Elsevier.

Wing JK (1990) SCAN: Schedules for Clinical Assessment in Neuropsychiatry. In: Stefanis CN (ed) Psychiatry. A world perspective. pp 85-90. Amsterdam: Elsevier.

Wing JK (1990) Introduction to the Field Trials of SCAN. In: Stefanis CN (ed) Psychiatry. A world perspective. pp 91-92. Amsterdam: Elsevier.

Wing JK (1991) Measuring and classifying clinical disorders. Learning from the PSE. In: Bebbington P (ed) Social psychiatry. Theory, methodology and practice. New Brunswick, NJ: Transaction.

Wing JK, Babor T, Brugha T, Burke J, Cooper J, Giel R, Jablensky A, Regier D and Sartorius N (1990) SCAN: Schedules for Clinical Assessment in Neuropsychiatry. Archives of General Psychiatry 47: 589-593.

Wing JK, Birley JLT, Cooper JE, Graham P and Isaacs AD (1967) Reliability of a procedure for measuring and classifying 'present psychiatric state'. British Journal of Psychiatry 113: 499-515.

Wing JK, Cooper JE and Sartorius N (1974) The description and classification of psychiatric symptoms. An instruction manual for the PSE and CATEGO system. London: Cambridge University Press.

Wing JK, Mann SA, Leff JP and Nixon JM (1978) The concept of a 'case' in psychiatric population surveys. Psychological Medicine 8: 203-217.

Wocjcik J, Gelenberg A, La Brie RA and Barg M (1980) Prevalence of tardive dyskinesia according to primary psychiatric diagnosis. Hillside Journal of Clinical Psychiatry 9: 3-11.

World Health Organization (1973) The International Pilot Study of Schizophrenia. Geneva: WHO.

World Health Organization (1991) International classification of diseases, tenth edition. Geneva: WHO.

Appendix:

This appendix contains a list of conditions in other chapters of ICD-10 that are often found in association with the disorders in Chapter V (F) itself. They are provided here so that psychiatrists recording diagnoses have the ICD terms and codes immediately to hand that will cover the most commonly associated diagnoses likely to be encountered in ordinary clinical practice. The majority of the conditions covered are given at the three-character level, but the four-character codes are given for a selection of those that will be used most frequently.

Chapter I: Certain infectious and parasitic diseases (A, B)
- A5   Congenital syphilis
  - .4 Late congenital neurosyphilis
- A52 Late syphilis
  - .1 Symptomatic neurosyphilis Includes: tabes dorsalis
- A81 Slow virus infections of central nervous system
  - .0 Creutzfeldt-Jakob disease
  - .1 Subacute sclerosing panencephalitis
- B22 Human immunodefciency virus (HIV) disease resulting in other specified diseases
  - .0 HIV disease resulting in encephalopathy (HIV dementia)

Chapter II: Neoplasms (C00 D48)
- C70 Malignant neoplasm of meninges
- C71 Malignant neoplasm of brain
- C72 Malignant neoplasm of spinal cord, cranial nerves and other parts of central nervous system
- D33 Benign neoplasm of brain and other parts of central nervous system
- D42 Neoplasm of uncertain and unknown behaviour of meninges
- D43 Neoplasm of uncertain and unknown behaviour of brain and central nervous system

Chapter IV: Endocrine, nutritional and metabolic diseases (E)
- E00 Congenital iodine-deficiency syndrome
- E01 Iodine-deficiency related thyroid disorders and allied conditions
- E02 Subclinical iodine-deficiency hypothyroidism
- E03 Other hypothyroidism
  - .2 Hypothyroidism due to medicaments and other exogenous substances
  - .5 Myxedema coma
- E05 Thyrotoxicosis (hyperthyroidism)
- E15 Nondiabetic hypoglycemic coma
- E22 Hyperfunction of pituitary gland
  - .0 Acromegaly and pituitary gigantism
  - .1 Hyperprolactinemia (includes drug-induced)
- E23 Hypofunction and other disorders of the pituitary gland
- E24 Cushing⁣s syndrome
- E30 Disorders of puberty, not elsewhere classified
  - .0 Delayed puberty
  - .1 Precocious puberty
- E34 Other endocrine disorders

.3   Short stature, not elsewhere classified
E51 Thiamin deficiency
    .2   Wernicke¡s encephalopathy
E54 Sequelae of malnutrition and other nutritional deficiencies
E66 Obesity
E70 Disorders of aromatic amino-acid metabolism
    .0   Classical phenylketonuria
E71 Disorders of branched-chain amino-acid metabolism and fatty acid metabolism
    .0   Maple-syrup-urine disease
E74 Other disorders of carbohydrate metabolism
E80 Disorders of porphyrin and bilirubin metabolism

Chapter VI: Diseases of the nervous system (G)
G00 Bacterial meningitis, not elsewhere classified. Includes: hemophilus, pneumococcal, streptococcal, staphylococcal and other bacterial meningitis
G01 Meningitis in bacterial diseases classified elsewhere. Includes: meningitis in: anthrax (A22.8+); gonococcal (A54.8+); leptospiral (A27.- +); listeriosis (A32.1+); Lyme disease (A69.2+); meningococcal (A39.0+); neurosyphilis (A52.1+); salmonella infection (A02.2+); syphilis, congenital (A50.4+); and secondary (A51.4+); tuberculous (A17.0+); typhoid fever (A01.- +)
G02 Meningitis in other infectious and parasitic diseases classified elsewhere
G03 Meningitis due to other and unspecified causes
G04 Encephalitis, myelitis and encephalomyelitis
G05 Encephalitis, myelitis and encephalomyelitis in diseases classified elsewhere. Includes: meningoencephalitis and meningomyelitis in infectious and parasitic diseases classified elsewhere
    .0   Encephalitis, myelitis and encephalomyelitis in bacterial diseases classified elsewhere. Includes: encephalitis in: listeriosis (A32.1+); Meningococcal syphilis (Congenital (A50.4+); and late (A52.1+); tuberculosis (A17.8+)
    .1   Encephalitis, myelitis and encephalomyelitis in viral diseases classified elsewhere. Includes: encephalitis in: adenovirus (A85.0+); cytomegaloviral (B25.8+); enteroviral (A85.0+); herpesviral (simplex) (B00.4+); influenza (J10.8+, J11.8+) measles (B05.0+); mumps (B26.2+) post chickenpox (B01.1+); rubella (B06.0+); zoster (B02.0+)
G06 Intracranial and intraspinal abscess and granuloma
    .2   Extradural and subdural abscess, unspecified
G10 Huntington¡s disease
G11 Hereditary ataxia and paraplegia
G20 Parkinson's disease
G21 Secondary Parkinsonism
    .0   Malignant neuroleptic syndrome
    .1   Other drug-induced secondary Parkinsonism
    .2   Secondary Parkinsonism due to other external agents
    .3   Postencephalitic Parkinsonism
G22 Parkinsonism in disease classified elsewhere
G24 Dystonia (includes dyskinesia)
    .0   Drug-induced dystonia

.3 Spasmodic torticollis

.8 Other dystonia. Includes: Tardive dyskinesia

G25 Other extrapyramidal and movement disorders. Includes: drug-induced tremor, myoclonus, chorea, tics; restless legs syndrome

G30 Alzheimer's disease

.0 Alzheimer's disease with early onset

.1 Alzheimer's disease with late onset

.8 Other Alzheimer's disease

.9 Alzheimer's disease, unspecified

G31 Other degenerative diseases of the nervous system, not elsewhere classified

.0 Circumscribed brain atrophy (Pick's disease)

.1 Senile degeneration of brain, not elsewhere classified

.2 Degeneration of the nervous system due to alcohol includes: alcoholic cerebellar ataxia and degeneration, cerebral degeneration and encephalopathy; dysfunction of the autonomic nervous system due to alcohol

.8 Other specified degenerative diseases of the nervous system. Includes: grey-matter degeneration; subacute necrotizing encephalopathy

.9 Degenerative disease of the nervous system, unspecified

G32 Other degenerative disorders of the nervous system in diseases classified elsewhere

G35 Multiple sclerosis

G37 Other demyelinating diseases of the central nervous system

.0 Diffuse sclerosis. Includes: periaxial encephalitis; Schilder's disease

G40 Epilepsy

.0 Localization-related (focal) (partial) idiopathic epilepsy and epileptic syndromes with seizures of localized onset. Includes: Benign childhood epilepsy with centrotemporal EEG spikes or occipital EEG paroxysms

.1 Localization-related (focal) (partial) symptomatic epilepsy and epileptic syndromes with simple partial seizures. Includes: attacks without alteration of consciousness

.2 Localization-related (focal) (partial) symptomatic epilepsy and epileptic syndromes with complex partial seizures. Includes: attacks with alteration of consciousness, often with automatisms

.3 Generalized idiopathic epilepsy and epileptic syndromes

.4 Other generalized epilepsy and epileptic syndromes. Includes: Salaam attacks

.5 Special epileptic syndromes. Includes: epileptic seizures related to alcohol, drugs and sleep deprivation

.6 Grand mal seizures, unspecified (with or without petit mal)

.7 Petit mal, unspecified, without grand mal seizures

G42 Status epilepticus

G43 Migraine

G44 Other headache syndromes

G45 Transient cerebral ischemic attacks and related syndromes

G46 Vascular syndromes of the brain in cerebrovascular diseases (I60 I67+)

G47 Sleep disorders

.4 Narcolepsy and cataplexy

G70 Myasthenia gravis and other myoneural disorders

.0　Myasthenia gravis
G91　Hydrocephalus
G92　Toxic encephalopathy
G93　Other disorders of brain
.1　Anoxic brain damage not elsewhere classified
.3　Postviral fatigue syndrome (Benign myalgic encephalomyelitis)
.4　Encephalopathy, unspecified
G97　Postprocedural disorders of the nervous system, not elsewhere classified
.0　Cerebrospinal fluid leak from spinal puncture

Chapter VII: Diseases of the eye and adnexa (H00 H59)
H40　Glaucoma
.6　Glaucoma secondary to drugs
H58　Other disorders of eye and adnexa in diseases classified elsewhere Includes: Argyll Robertson phenomenon or pupil, syphilitic (A52.1+)

Chapter VIII: Diseases of the ear and mastoid process (H60 H95)
H93　Other disorders of ear, not elsewhere classified
.1　Tinnitus

Chapter IX: Diseases of the circulatory system (I)
I10　Essential (primary) hypertension
I60　Subarachnoid hemorrhage
I61　Intracerebral hemorrhage
I62　Other nontraumatic intracranial hemorrhage
.0　Subdural hemorrhage (nontraumatic)
.1　Extradural hemorrhage (nontraumatic)
I63　Cerebral infarction
I64　Stroke, not specified as hemorrhage or infarction
I65　Occlusion and stenosis of precerebral arteries, not resulting in cerebral infarction
I66　Occlusion and stenosis of cerebral arteries, not resulting in cerebral infarction
I67　Other cerebrovascular diseases
.2 Cerebral atherosclerosis
.3 Progressive vascular leukoencephalopathy (Binswanger's disease)
.4 Hypertensive encephalopathy
I68　Cerebrovascular involvement in diseases classified elsewhere
.0 Cerebral amyloid angiopathy (E85)
I69　Sequelae of cerebrovascular disease
I95　Hypotension
.2 Hypotension due to drugs

Chapter X: Diseases of the respiratory system (J)
J10　Influenza due to identified influenza virus
.8 Influenza with other manifestations, influenza virus identified
J11　Influenza, virus not identified
.8 Influenza with other manifestations, virus not identified

J42 Unspecified chronic bronchitis
J43 Emphysema
J45 Asthma

Chapter XI: Diseases of the digestive system (K)
K25 Gastric ulcer
K26 Duodenal ulcer
K27 Peptic ulcer, site unspecified
K29 Gastritis and duodenitis
    .2 Alcoholic gastritis
K30 Dyspepsia
K58 Irritable bowel syndrome
K59 Other functional intestinal disorders
K70 Alcoholic liver disease
K71 Toxic liver disease. Includes: drug-induced liver disease
K86 Other diseases of pancreas
    .0 Alcohol-induced chronic pancreatitis

Chapter XII: Diseases of the skin and subcutaneous tissue (L)
L20 Atopic dermatitis
L98 Other disorders of the skin and subcutaneous tissue, not elsewhere classified
    .1 Factitial dermatitis. Includes: neurotic excoriation

Chapter XIII: Diseases of the musculoskeletal system and connective tissue (M)
M32 Systemic lupus erythematosus
M54 Dorsalgia

Chapter XIV: Diseases of the genitourinary system (N)
N48 Other disorders of penis
    .3 Priapism
    .4 Impotence of organic origin
N91 Absent, scanty and rare menstruation
N94 Pain and other conditions associated with female genital organs and menstrual cycle
    .3 Premenstrual tension syndrome
    .4 Primary dysmenorrhoea
    .5 Secondary dysmenorrhoea
    .6 Dysmenorrhoea, unspecified
N95 Menopausal and other perimenopausal disorders
    .1 Menopausal or female climacteric states
    .3 States associated with artificial menopause

Chapter XV: Pregnancy, childbirth and the puerperium (O)
O04 Medical abortion
O35 Maternal care for known or suspected fetal abnormality and damage
    .4 Maternal care for (suspected) damage to fetus from alcohol
    .5 Maternal care for (suspected) damage to fetus by drugs (from drug addiction)

O99 Other maternal diseases classifiable elsewhere but complicating pregnancy, childbirth and the puerperium

.3 Mental disorders and diseases of the nervous system, complicating pregnancy, childbirth and the puerperium Conditions in F00 F99 and G00 G99

Chapter XVII: Congenital malformations, deformations, and chromosomal abnormalities (Q)

Q02 Microcephaly

Q03 Congenital hydrocephalus

Q04 Other congenital malformations of brain

Q05 Spina bifida

Q75 Other congenital malformations of skull and face bones

Q85 Phakomatoses, not elsewhere classified

.0 Neurofibromatosis (nonmalignant)

.1 Tuberous sclerosis

Q86 Congenital malformation syndromes due to known exogenous causes, not elsewhere classified

.0 Fetal alcohol syndrome (dysmorphic)

Q90 Down's syndrome

.0 Trisomy 21, meiotic nondisjunction

.1 Trisomy 21, mosaicism (mitotic nondisjunction)

.2 Trisomy 21, translocation

.9 Down's syndrome, unspecified

Q91 Edwards' syndrome and Patau's syndrome

Q93 Monosomies and deletions from the autosomes, not elsewhere classified

.4 Deletion of short arm of chromosomes (Cri-du-chat syndrome)

Q96 Turner's syndrome

Q97 Other sex chromosome abnormalities, female phenotype, not elsewhere classified

.0 Klinefelter's syndrome karyotype 47, XXX

.1 Klinefelter's syndrome, male with more than two X chromosomes

.2 Klinefelter's syndrome, Male with 46, XX karyotype

.4 Klinefelter's syndrome, unspecified

Q99 Other chromosome abnormality NEC

Chapter XVIII: Symptoms, signs, abnormal clinical and laboratory. Findings not elsewhere classified (R)

R55 Syncope and collapse

R56 Convulsions, not elsewhere classified

.0 Febrile convulsions

.8 Other and unspecified convulsions

R62 Lack of expected normal physiological development

.0 Delayed milestone

.8 Other lack of expected normal physiological development

.9 Lack of expected normal physiological development, unspecified

R63 Symptoms and signs concerning food and fluid intake

.0 Anorexia

.1 Polydipsia

.4 Abnormal weight loss

.5 Abnormal weight gain

R78 Findings of drugs and other substances normally not found in blood. Includes: alcohol (.0); opiate drug (.1); cocaine (.2); hallucinogen (.3); other drugs of addictive potential (.4); psychotropic drug (.5); abnormal level of lithium (.8)

R83 Abnormal findings in cerebrospinal fluid

R90 Abnormal findings on diagnostic imaging of central nervous system

R94 Abnormal results of function studies

.0 Abnormal results of function studies of central nervous system Includes: abnormal electroencephalogram [EEG]

Chapter XIX: Injury, poisoning and certain other consequences of external causes (S,T)

S06 Intracranial injury

.0 Concussion

.1 Traumatic cerebral oedema

.2 Diffuse brain injury

.3 Focal brain injury

.4 Epidural hemorrhage

.5 Traumatic subdural hemorrhage

.6 Traumatic subarachnoid hemorrhage

.7 Intracranial injury with prolonged coma

Chapter XX: External causes of morbidity and mortality (V, W, X, Y) Intentional self-harm (X60 X84) Includes purposely self-inflicted self harm and suicide

X60 Intentional self-poisoning by and exposure to non-narcotic analgesics, antipyretics and antirheumatic

X61 Intentional self-poisoning by and exposure to antiepileptics, sedative-hypnotics, antiparkinson and psychotropic drugs, not elsewhere classified Includes: antidepressants; barbiturates; neuroleptics [tranquillizers]; psychostimulants

X62 Intentional self-poisoning by and exposure to narcotics and psychodysleptics, not elsewhere classified Includes: cannabis (derivatives); cocaine; codeine, heroin; LSD; mescaline; methadone; morphine; opium (alkaloids)

X63 Intentional self-poisoning by and exposure to other drugs acting on the autonomic nervous systems

X64 Intentional self-poisoning by and exposure to other and unspecified drugs and biological substances

X65 Intentional self-poisoning by alcohol

X66 Intentional self-poisoning by organic solvents and halogenated hydrocarbons and their vapors

X67 Intentional self-poisoning by other gases and vapors Includes: corrosive aromatics, acids and caustic alkalis

X68 Intentional self-poisoning by pesticides

X69 Intentional self-poisoning by other and unspecified chemicals and noxious substances Includes: corrosive aromatics, acids and caustic alkalis

X70 Intentional self-harm by hanging, strangulation and suffocation

X71 Intentional self-harm by drowning and submersion

X72 Intentional self-harm by handgun discharge

X73 Intentional self-harm by rifle, shotgun and larger firearm discharge
X74 Intentional self-harm by other and unspecified firearm discharge
X75 Intentional self-harm by explosive material
X76 Intentional self-harm by fire and flames
X77 Intentional self-harm by steam, hot vapors and hot objects
X78 Intentional self-harm by sharp object
X79 Intentional self-harm by blunt object
X80 Intentional self-harm by jumping from a high place
X81 Intentional self-harm by jumping or lying before moving object
X82 Intentional self-harm by crashing of motor vehicle
X83 Intentional self-harm by other specified means Includes: crashing of aircraft; electrocution; extremes of cold
X84 Intentional self-harm by unspecified means Assault (X85 Y09) Includes: homicide and injuries inflicted by another person with intent to injure or kill, by any means
X93 Assault by handgun discharge
X99 Assault by sharp object
Y00 Assault by blunt object
Y04 Assault by bodily force
Y05 Sexual assault by bodily force
Y06 Neglect and abandonment
Y07 Other maltreatment syndromes Includes: mental cruelty; physical abuse; sexual abuse; torture
Drugs and biological substances causing adverse effects in therapeutic use (Y40 Y59)
Y46 Antiepileptics and anti-Parkinsonism drugs
   .7   Anti-Parkinsonism drugs
Y47 Sedatives, hypnotics and antianxiety drugs
Y49 Psychotropic drugs, not elsewhere classified
   .0   Tricyclic and tetracyclic antidepressants
   .1   Monoamine-oxidase inhibitor antidepressants
   .2   Other and unspecified antidepressants
   .3   Phenothiazine antipsychotics and neuroleptics
   .4   Butyrophenone and thiothixene neuroleptics
   .5   Other antipsychotics and neuroleptics
   .6   Psychodysleptics [hallucinogens]
   .7   Psychostimulants with abuse potential
   .8   Other psychotropic agents, not elsewhere classified
   .9   Psychotropic drug, unspecified
Y50 Central nervous system stimulants, not elsewhere classified
Y51 Drugs primarily affecting the autonomic nervous system
Y57 Other and unspecified drugs and medicaments

Chapter XXI: Factors influencing health status and contact with health services (Z)
Z00 General examination and investigation of persons without complaint and reported diagnosis
   .4   General psychiatric examination, not elsewhere classified
Z02 Examination and encounter for administrative purposes
   .3   Examination for recruitment to armed forces
   .4   Examination for driving license

.6   Examination for insurance purposes

.7   Issue of medical certificate

Z03 Medical observation and evaluation for suspected diseases and conditions

    .2   Observation for suspected mental and behavioural disorders. Includes: observation for dissocial behaviour, fire-setting, gang activity, and shop lifting, without manifest psychiatric behaviour

Z04 Examination and observation for other reasons. Includes: examination for medicolegal reasons

    .6   General psychiatric examination, requested by authority

Z50 Care involving use of rehabilitation procedures

    .2   Alcohol rehabilitation

    .3   Drug rehabilitation

    .4   Psychotherapy, not elsewhere classified

    .7   Occupational therapy and vocational rehabilitation, not elsewhere classified

    .8   Care involving use of other specified rehabilitation procedures Includes: tobacco abuse rehabilitation, training in activities of daily living [ADL]

Z54 Convalescence

    .3   Convalescence following psychotherapy

Z55 Problems related to education and literacy

Z56 Problems related to employment and unemployment

Z59 Problems related to housing and economic circumstances

Z60 Problems related to social environment

    .0   Problems of adjustment to life-cycle transitions

    .1   Atypical parenting situation

    .2   Living alone

    .3   Acculturation difficulty

    .4   Social exclusion and rejection

    .5   Target of perceived adverse discrimination and persecutions

    .8   Other specified problems related to social environment

Z61 Problems related to negative life events in childhood

    .0   Loss of love relationship in childhood

    .1   Removal from home in childhood

    .2   Altered pattern of family relationships in childhood

    .3   Events resulting in loss of self esteem in childhood

    .4   Problems related to alleged sexual abuse of child by person within primary support group

    .5   Problems related to alleged sexual abuse of child by person outside of primary support group

    .6   Problems related to alleged physical child abuse

    .7   Personal frightening experience in childhood

    .8   Other negative life events in childhood

Z62 Other problems related to upbringing

    .0   Inadequate parental supervision and control

    .1   Parental overprotection

    .2   Institutional upbringing

    .3   Hostility towards and scapegoating of child

    .4   Emotional neglect of child

.5 Other problems related to neglect in upbringing

.6 Inappropriate parental pressures and other abnormal qualities of upbringing

.8 Other specified problems related to upbringing

Z63 Other problems related to primary support group, including family circumstances

.0 Problems in relationship with spouse or partner

.1 Problems in relationship with parents and in-laws

.2 Inadequate family support

.3 Absence of family member

.4 Disappearance or death of family member

.5 Disruption of family by separation or divorce

.6 Dependent relative needing care at home

.7 Other stressful life events affecting family and household

.8 Other specified problems related to primary group

Z64 Problems related to certain psychological circumstances

.0 Problems related to unwanted pregnancy

.2 Seeking and accepting physical, nutritional and chemical interventions known to be hazardous and harmful

.3 Seeking and accepting behavioural and psychological interventions known to be hazardous and harmful

.4 Discord with counsellors. Includes: probation officer; social worker

Z65 Problems related to other psychological circumstances

.0 Conviction in civil and criminal proceedings without imprisonment

.1 Imprisonment ant other incarceration

.2 Problems related to release from prison

.3 Problems related to other legal circumstances. Includes: arrest; child custody or support proceedings

.4 Victim of crime and terrorism (including torture)

Z70 Counselling related to sexual attitude, behaviour and orientation

Z71 Persons encountering health services for other counselling and medical advice, not elsewhere classified

.4 Alcohol abuse counselling and surveillance

.5 Drug abuse counselling and surveillance

.6 Tobacco abuse counselling

Z72 Problems relating to lifestyle

.0 Tobacco use

.1 Alcohol use

.2 Drug use

.3 Lack of physical exercise

.4 Inappropriate diet or eating habits

.5 High risk sexual behaviour

.6 Gambling and betting

.8 Other problems related to lifestyle Includes: self-damaging behaviour

Z73 Problems related to life-management difficulty

.0 Burn-out

.1 Accentuation of personality traits. Includes: Type A behaviour pattern

.2 Lack of relaxation or leisure

    .3   Stress, not elsewhere classified
    .4   Inadequate social skills, not elsewhere classified
    .5   Social role conflict, not elsewhere classified
Z75 Problems related to medical facilities and other health care
    .1   Person awaiting admission to adequate facility elsewhere
    .2   Other waiting period for an investigation and treatment
    .5   Holiday relief care
Z76 Persons encountering health services in other circumstances
    .0   Issue of repeat prescription
    .5   Malingerer [conscious simulation]

WHO designated SCAN Training and Reference Centers

Aarhus
Dr Aksel Bertelsen
WHO Collaborating Centre for Research
and Training in Mental Health
Institute of Psychiatric Demography
Aarhus Psychiatric Hospital
DK-8240 Risskov
Denmark
Tel: 45 86 17 77 77
Fax: 45 86 17 74 55
Language: Danish
Status: TRC

Ankara
Dr A. Gvüs
Dept. of Psychiatry
Hacettepe University
Ankara
Turkey
Tel: 90 4 310 8693
Fax: 90 4 310 1938
Language: Turkish
Status: TRC

Bangalore
Dr. Somnath Chatterji
National Institute of Mental
Health and Neurosciences
Department of Psychiatry
Post Bag No 2979
Bangalore 560029
India
Tel: 91 80 64 21 21 x 221
Tel: 91 80 64 80 73 (home)
Fax: 91 80 66 31 830
e-mail: nimhans!root@vigyan.iisc.ernet.in
Language: Hindi/Kannada
Status: TRC

Beijing
Professor Shen Yucun
Institute of Mental Health
Beijing Medical College
Beijing 100083
China (People's Republic of)
Tel: 86 1 440 531 (318)
Fax: 86 1 202 7314
Language: Chinese
Status: TRC

Groningen
Professor R. Giel
& Dr Niekenhaus
Department of Social Psychiatry
Academisch Ziekenhuis
Postbus 30.001, Oostersingel 59
9700 RB Groningen
The Netherlands
Tel: 31 50 61 38 37
Fax: 31 50 34 59 15
Language: Dutch
Status: TRC

German Joint Training and Reference Centres

Lübeck
Professor H. Dilling
Klinik für Psychiatrie der Medizinische Hochschule
Ratzeburger Allee 160
2400 Lübeck 1
Germany
Tel: 49 451 500 2440
Fax: 49 451 500 2603
Language: German
Status: GER-TRC

Mannheim
Professor H. Hdfner
& Dr K. Maurer
Zentralinstitut für seelische Gesundheit
Quadrat J.5
Postfach 5970
6800 Mannheim 1
Germany
Tel: 49 621 1703 738
Fax: 49 621 234 29
Language: German
Status: GER-TRC

Greece
Dr. V.G. Mavreas
University Research Institute
of Mental Health
Eginition Hospital
74, Vas. Sophias Avenue
11528 Athens
Greece
Tel: 30 1 724 7618
Fax: 30 1 724 3905
Language: Greek
Status: TRC

Luxembourg
Professor Charles Pull
Centre hospitalier de Luxembourg
Service de Neuropsychiatrie
4, rue Barbli
Luxembourg
Tel: 352 4411-2256
Fax: 352 458 762
Language: French
Status: TRC

Nagasaki
Professor Y. Nakane
Department of Neuro Psychiatry
University of Nagasaki
7-1, Sakomoto-Machi
Nagasaki 852
Japan
Tel: 81 958 47 21 11 ext 2860
Fax: 81 958 49 43 72
Language: Japanese
Status: TRC

Santandar
Professor J.L. Vazquez-Barquero
Unidad de Investigacion en
Psiquiatria Social de Cantabria
Hospital Universitario
"Marques de Valdecilla"
Av Valdecilla S/N
39008 Santandar
Spain
Tel: 34 42 202 520 ext 72545
Tel: 34 42 202 545 direct
Fax: 34 42 202 655
Language: Spanish
Status: TRC

Sao Paulo
Dr. F. Lotufo Neto
Dr. L.Andrade
Hospital das Clinicas
Faculdade de Medicina da
Universidade de Sao Paulo
Caixa Postal 8091
Sao Paulo
Brazil
Tel: 55 11 210 4311
Fax:
Language: Portuguese
Status: TRC

United Kingdom Joint Training and Reference Centres

London
Professor John Wing
The Royal College of Psychiatrists
Research Unit
11 Grosvenor Crescent
London SW1X 7EE
United Kingdom
Tel: 44 71 235 2996
Fax: 44 71 235 2954
Language: English
Status: UK-TRC
            Coordinator

London
Dr. Paul Bebbington
MRC Social Psychiatry Unit
Institute of Psychiatry
De Crespigny Park
London SE5 8AF
UK
Tel: 44 71 703 5411
Tel: 44 71 919 3497 (direct)
Fax: 44 71 703 0458
Language: English
Status: UK-TRC
            Secretary

Leicester
Dr. Terry Brugha
Department of Psychiatry
University of Leicester
Leicester Royal Infirmary
PO Box 65
Leicester LE2 7LX
UK
Tel: 44 535 523 246
Fax: 44 535 523 293
Language: English
Status: UK-TRC

Manchester
Dr Louis Appleby
Senior Lecturer
University of Manchester
Dept of Psychiatry
Withington Hospital
West Didsbury
Manchester M20 8LR
United Kingdom
Tel: 44 61 447 4354
Fax: 44 61 445 9263
Language: English
Status: UK-TRC

Nottingham
Dr. Glynn Harrison
Professorial Unit
Mapperley Hospital
Porchester Road
Nottingham NG3 6AA
United Kingdom
Tel: 44 602 691 300 x40681
Fax: 44 602 856 396
e-mail: G.Harrison@vme.ccc.nottingham.ac.uk
Language: English
Status: UK-TRC

United States Joint Training and Reference Centres

Baltimore

Dr. A. Tien
The John Hopkins University
School of Hygiene and Public Health
Department of Mental Hygiene
624 North Broadway
Baltimore, Maryland 21205
USA
Tel: 1 410 955 1709
Fax: 1 410 955 9088
e-mail: allen@atien.sph.jhu.edu
Language: English
Status: US-TRC

Dr. A. Romanoski
The Johns Hopkins Hospital
Meyer Building
Room 4-119
600 N Wolfe Street
Baltimore, Maryland, 21287-7419
USA
Tel: 1 410 955 7011
Fax: 1 410 955 0946
Language: English
Status: US-TRC

Farmington
Dr J. Escobar
& Dr T. Babor
School of Medicine
Department of Psychiatry
University of Connecticut Health Centre
Farmington CT 06032
USA
Tel: 1 203 679 3423
Fax: 1 203 679 1296
Language: English
Status: US-TRC

St Louis
Dr Wilson M. Compton III
Department of Psychiatry
Washington University
School of Medicine
4940 Children's Place
St. Louis, Missouri 63110
USA
Tel: 1 314 362 2413
Fax: 1 314 362 4294
e-mail: compton@epi.wustl.edu
Language: English
Status: US-TRC

SCAN Field Trial Centres

Cardiff
Dr Anne Farmer
Department of Psychological
Medicine
University of Wales
Health Park
Cardiff CF4 4XN WALES
United Kingdom
Tel: 44 222 755 944 ext. 3241
Fax:
Language: English
Status: FTC

Geneva
Dr L. Barrelet
Clinique Psychiatrie Cantonal
2018 Perreux
Switzerland
Tel: 038 44 11 11
Fax: 038 42 64 76
Language: French
Status: FTC